WHY?

The Question that Could Save Your Life

A Guide to Taking Control of
Your Health and Health Care

ROBERT BROWN, DDS

TRIMARK PRESS, INC.
368 S. MILITARY TRAIL
DEERFIELD BEACH, FL 33442
800.889.0693
WWW.TRIMARKPRESS.COM

D0041830

LIBRARY OF CONGRESS CATALOGING-IN-PUBLICATION DATA

WHY? THE QUESTION THAT COULD SAVE YOUR LIFE
A GUIDE TO TAKING CONTROL OF YOUR HEALTH AND HEALTH CARE

ROBERT J. BROWN, DDS

P. CM.
ISBN: 978-0-9904211-7-7
LIBRARY OF CONGRESS CONTROL NUMBER: 2014949184

H14
10 9 8 7 6 5 4 3 2 1
SECOND EDITION
PRINTED AND BOUND IN THE UNITED STATES OF AMERICA

WWW.DRBROWNWHY.COM

*trimark*press

A PUBLICATION OF TRIMARK PRESS, INC.
368 SOUTH MILITARY TRAIL
DEERFIELD BEACH, FL 33442
800.889.0693
WWW.TRIMARKPRESS.COM

For Carol Brown
1953 - 2011

*To my gift from God, Carol Kidwell Brown, the most
wonderful person I have ever known. In spite of her
suffering, she was almost always positive and uplifting,
able to get a whole roomful of her friends laughing, so
kind and generous. Carol, we all miss you, and I will
always love you. May this book prevent needless
suffering for all who read it and more.*

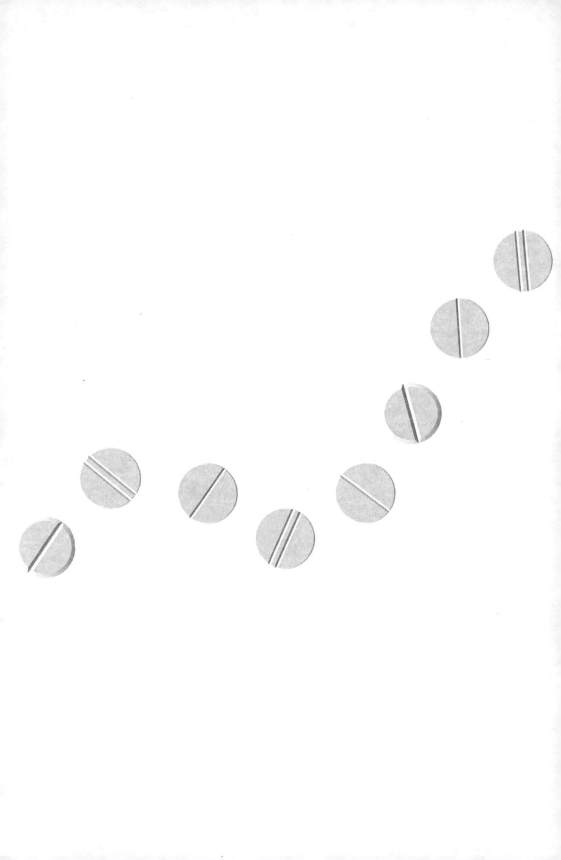

CONTENTS

TABLE OF CONTENTS

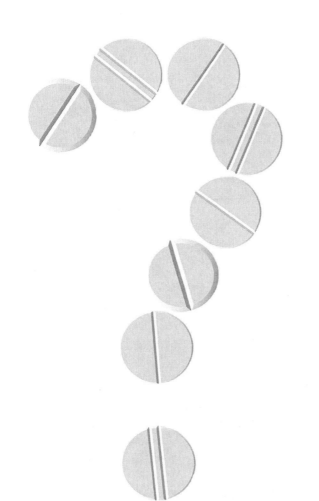

PREFACE

Preface

Throughout my life as a medical professional, I have noticed that most doctors never ask the most important question about their patients' symptoms: *Why?* They have been taught that x + y = z—and anything that doesn't readily conform to established medical protocols and beliefs isn't recognized as worth considering.

But as a doctor, I always knew that I needed to go deeper. And at three significant times in my life, both loved ones and I were able to reap the benefits of this realization. Let me share with you the stories of what happened—they are the reason for this book.

• • •

In my early childhood, I loved growing my own veggies. I would eat onions like apples, and I loved everything we grew. One day when I was seven, I was enjoying my normal Saturday playing with my vegetables (I never considered it work). We lived in the Berkeley Hills, and the neighbor who lived uphill from my garden apparently had parked his car and not set the parking brake. Sitting in the garden, I turned to see a bumper about to hit me in the head. The next thing I remember, clear to this day, is looking up at light coming through the floorboards as the car ran over me.

It was 1945, and the hospital was full of war victims. I will never forget the moaning of all the wounded soldiers, which kept me awake that night. Fortunately, I was treated quickly and released the next day. I recovered well, seemed to be free of complications, and went on to live a very active, athletic childhood.

Off and on through my teens, however, I had pain in my left abdomen—but no one was able to diagnose it. At the University of California at Berkeley, I was hospitalized with the pain and was told it was psychosomatic. When I was thirty-one, the pain got out of control, and this time, it was diagnosed as diverticulitis—something like appendicitis but on the left side. A hideously painful air-contrast barium study was done, which revealed that my left colon had been crushed. That was where the car tire had gone over me.

A left colectomy was performed when I was thirty-two. I was recovering well after the surgery, but then the surgeon neglected to review my history and prescribed an antibiotic that had previously been shown to be ineffective at controlling the existing infection; the bacteria in my intestine were resistant to this antibiotic. This would not be his last mistake—but it was a doozy.

Infection of my entire abdomen (peritonitis) set in, and I went into a coma, with a fever reaching 105+ degrees. While in the coma, I died. And like others who've had near-death experiences (NDEs), I went through the tunnel with the light and heaven at the end.

Also like others', mine was a beautiful experience in which I was informed that it was not my time and that I had very important things to accomplish. I was sent back into my body and woke up demanding the antibiotic that would save my life. Thank God I had studied pharmacology! Within thirty minutes of having an IV of chloramphenicol, I knew I was going to survive. I had been in the coma for six days.

Once I was past the critical stage, the pain in my gut was so intense that I couldn't eat. I was taken to radiology on a cold gurney, where I was x-rayed for hours. If it hadn't been for one of my patients, a volunteer at the hospital, seeing me there and bringing me warm blanket-sheets, I would have been left to suffer—I was too sick to complain.

The "specialists" finally came up with a diagnosis: a pancreatic cyst. I was not supposed to have any fat in my diet, so that food could by-pass the cyst. I was eventually able to eat some food, and while it was painful, once the food got past the cyst, I would start to feel better.

I decided to go to Hawaii to recover, but once again, I ended up in the hospital because of the pain of trying to eat. I had to keep eating. I had lost forty pounds and felt as if I were starving. Then one evening, while having dinner at the Plantation Garden Inn in Kauai, I ordered a creamy banana-rum drink—and had dinner with no pain for the first time.

I made my own diagnosis: it was a peritoneal cyst. So logical! I had peritonitis, and my body had walled it off to form a cyst the size of an orange right on my duodenum (stomach outlet).

The cream in the drink had caused the duodenal sphincter to close, slowing down the food leaving my stomach and allowing me to eat without pain.

Two specialists who really had not understood physiology had misdiagnosed my disease. Worse than that, they had not even followed up to see if their treatment plan was working. I took over my own treatment from then on and not only got well, but so well that I was able to become athletic again.

My experience with God changed my life forever. Then, five years after my NDE, I had a visitation of sorts, in which the implications of the entire occurrence were reinforced and made extremely clear. What if I hadn't been a physiologist with medical training? I probably wouldn't be here writing about what I've learned.

As I look back on my life, there were a lot of whys that were never asked and doctors who were so devoted to their specialty that they were blind to the real cause of my symptoms.

This is the reason I'm going to attempt to make it possible for the average person without medical training to be able to understand a holistic approach to his or her health. There's a big difference between being treated by the medical books and the pharmaceutical industry and being treated by a practitioner who is humble enough to really care and ask *why*. The latter is a person who can get "outside the box"—much to his or her patient's good fortune.

• • •

My second story happened on a beautiful day in July 1977. My daughter, Michelle, was two years old—a wonderful, active child. My wife, Carol, had placed bells on Michelle's shoes to track her location within our home. Everything seemed normal, when suddenly, there was silence—no bell sound to catch Carol's attention.

Rushing to see why, Carol found Michelle unconscious and gasping for air. Immediately, we were off to the doctor with the baby. It was quicker for us to drive than to call 911, and I had worked at a hospital while in school and had a lot of emergency training.

Our physician said it was asthma and referred us to a pediatric allergist. He wrote the prescriptions and told us this disease would probably always have to be dealt with—our adored little girl was possibly compromised for life. Sadly, we returned home, emotionally wiped out.

Over the next few months, we gave Michelle the prescribed asthma medicines, which kept the disease under control. She hated the meds, though, because they were adrenaline-like and they uncomfortably elevated her energy. She would cry whenever it was time to take them.

Finally, I had had enough—I hit the books. As I studied Michelle's current method of drug treatment, I could see many possible future problems. Long-term use of steroids can lead to Addison's disease, for example, and the terrible symptoms associated with it.

A few years before, I had attended a dental-society meeting where an oral surgeon had spoken about his sister being cured of the asthma that was killing her. I was so intrigued that I took the speaker to lunch to learn more.

The surgeon was leaving his practice to begin a holistic clinic in Idaho with another doctor. He was so impressed by alternative medicine that he had become committed to it.

Inspired by that incident, I began my study of alternative medicine, seeking answers to the question, why does asthma exist? I also asked myself why it was necessary to drug the patient to cover the symptoms. I believed that with the Western approach of curing all with drugs, it was likely that, even if Michelle didn't die, she would definitely not be healthy.

Realizing that asthma is most likely a severe allergic reaction to something, possibly a food, I found a book entitled *The Pulse Test* by Arthur Coca. Using his methods, I tested Michelle to find she had three serious food allergies: to wheat, milk, and peanuts.

We eliminated these food groups from her diet, and thirty-six years later, she runs a physical-fitness business—and is a martial arts world champion.

• • •

Here's the third story I want to share with you. We were at Squaw Valley in California with our friends Perry and Carl. The snow was perfect, and the skiing was great, with no long lines at the chairlifts. Perry was lagging behind, and Carol stopped by the Headwall Chair to wait for her. I stopped about 100 yards ahead.

As I looked back to see where she was, I

watched in horror as a speeding skier lost control, becoming airborne and hitting Carol in the legs. Carol flew through the air like a rag doll, and by the time I made it up the hill to her, she was just coming to. Both her legs were broken— the right lower leg in many places.

I was thankful the skier didn't hit higher on Carol's body. But the incident began over ten years of suffering through thirty surgeries, most of them due to medical mistakes. The first ortho-pedic surgeon attempted four surgeries, each failing to close the wound on the most injured leg. They began to talk about amputation; this time I asked *why.*

Their answer was that the blood reaching the area was not oxygenated enough to resist infection and create healing. I suggested hyperbaric oxygen. The leg was saved.

The local surgeons referred her to the best trauma orthopedic surgeon, who taught at the University of California, Davis. Dr. C. brought in his students to show them what not to do when a lower leg has several fractures. A procedure called "external fixation" was then used, and the wound was left open to heal from the inside so that plastic surgery could finally cover it.

Now enter two plastic surgeons who tried three surgeries, only to fail again. Not only did they not understand the physiology of this type of wound healing, but they had no idea how to control the incredible pain Carol was experiencing.

After Carol had suffered for several days, with the physicians thinking she had a drug problem, I found a friend who specialized in pain management. Within hours, Carol was practically pain-free. Instead of faulting the patient, the pain specialist looked into why the pain was out of control—and addressed the problem.

What causes pain after such traumatic surgery is swelling, inflammation, and the trauma of surgery itself. The pain specialist controlled the swelling with a diuretic, the inflammation with an anti-inflammatory, and the pain with a stronger, orally administered narcotic. (The oral administration maintains a more level control of pain, preventing spiking.)

The *next why* Carol's MDs didn't ask was *why* the wound wouldn't close. So I began researching and found the best doctor in the field. He informed us that without *periosteum*—the membrane that covers bone—and adequate blood supply, proper healing of the bone could not take place. To bring blood to the area, it was necessary to transplant a muscle from her abdomen, along with its artery and vein—a complex surgery of seven hours.

Twenty-two days later, we left the hospital, with the leg still attached to Carol and the wound closed for the first time in years.

It would seem that should be the end of the story, but there's more—lots more mistakes that would go on for years.

• • •

As I look back, it appears that medicine is so specialized that one specialty doesn't understand the other, and very few specialties have a working knowledge of the basic sciences, such as physiology, pain management, infection control, and pharmacology.

It seems there is so much emphasis in a doctor's training on memorizing standard practices of medicine, a left-brain function, that right-brain function is diminished or lost. Yet the right brain is what makes it possible to think "outside the box." Unfortunately, right-brained thinking seems to be the enemy of many teachers and professors. If you're in a college class and think outside the box, you can flunk. We'll look closer at this serious problem in chapter 1.

But my purpose for this book is to show you why our current system doesn't work. If we understand the significance of asking *why*, then we have a chance to make a difference in our lives and those of our families: the difference between living a life of pain and suffering and living one of joy and good health.

I believe that anyone who is willing to look beyond the standard way of approaching health and medicine can find, as I have, a new lease on life. Thank you for joining me in my journey to change the way we look at health care so that we can change the paradigm of what we call our "health-care" system and enjoy life well into our senior years.

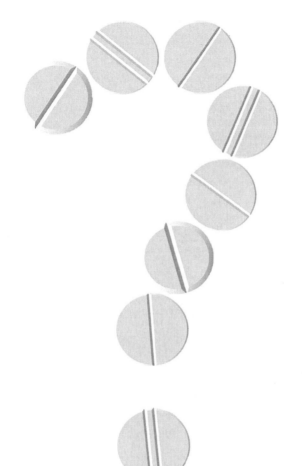

ACKNOWLEDGMENTS

ACKNOWLEDGMENTS

With gratitude I acknowledge the many patients who have followed my advice and achieved new health. That is what inspires me to continue learning and to not want to retire.

To a professor of undergraduate chemistry who, even though I earned it, would not give me an A in a 5-unit course—thank you. This grade would have put me in dental school one year earlier. His reason for not giving me an A was that one more year of physiology would be of great value to me and my career. I thank him because that extra year turned out to be invaluable.

To all my friends and colleagues who have begged me to write this book, thank you.

To those "outside the box" professors and professionals who have led me to believe there is hope to change the system, thank you.

To my editor, Jennifer Read Hawthorne,

whose patience, knowledge, and expertise were absolutely invaluable to me in completing this endeavor, thank you.

To you, the reader, for seeking this knowledge and, hopefully, doing what you can to help, thank you.

I thank you all.

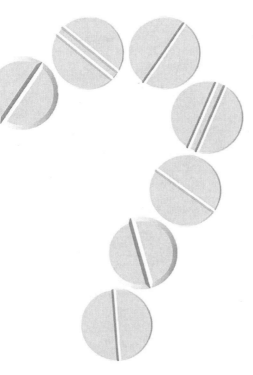

INTRODUCTION

INTRODUCTION

Just yesterday I was at the gas station waiting in line to buy bottled water. I watched the man ahead of me pay for four bags of chocolate chip cookies and a pack of cigarettes. He was probably in his fifties but would likely be perceived by most as a man in his seventies. Deep inside, I knew he knew better, but he just didn't care.

By this time, I was already into the seventh chapter of this book, but I realized that I had better introduce the reader to the frustrations of most doctors, particularly those in alternative medicine.

Immediate gratification, with little or no responsibility for the results, seems to be more the rule in society today than the exception. With all the information available about how to live a healthy life, you'd think people would hesitate to knowingly destroy their health. But it's just not the case. It's so easy to put off till tomorrow those habits that improve one's health and vitality—until, all of a sudden, tomorrow is here and you're miserable and wish you could go back and take care of yourself.

And unfortunately, it's truly the majority of us that suffer the results of self-neglect, often not realizing it until it's too late to stop the decay and disease. I wish everyone could have a visit from the Ghost of Christmas Yet to Come in Dickens's *A Christmas Carol*. If only we could see ourselves in the future, viewing the results of our good habits versus the bad ones we indulge in!

Actually, this movie is available to us: a trip to any retirement community will do. Check out the eighty-plus-year-old men and women playing golf. Then go inside to see the seventy-year-old men and women having to be assisted, unable to walk.

Which would you like to be? Ask that of yourself as you raise that donut to your mouth and follow it with orange juice or, even better, an energy drink for breakfast. Next, french fries, a Big Mac, and a Coke for lunch. Then, pizza with a beer for dinner.

For those of us in medicine and dentistry who try to make up for such poor eating habits, it can be so frustrating that many just give up and treat the symptoms. But I have come to the point that, if patients won't commit to helping themselves, I refer them to another practice that specializes in treating symptoms. Such patients love the instant gratification of drugs, which let them carry on with their horrible habits of more instant gratification through eating unhealthy food, drinking liquor, and indulging in other bad habits.

Then there are the opinions from those who never want to change. And then there's the concept of "evidence-based" medicine, used in all fields of medicine and dentistry, which holds that if a practitioner cannot show accepted scientific evidence in favor of his procedure or treatment plan, it should not be allowed. Where does the evidence for anything new and different come from if someone does not first get "outside the box"?

"Evidence-based" medicine is nebulous, at best. Does the evidence have to come only from institutions someone deems worthy to agree with? Why can't hundreds or thousands of years of the successful practice of a procedure using certain natural remedies be enough to allow for the procedure's use?

And what about the food we eat and its relationship to our health? In my experience, following the Paleo Diet is the best way of emulating what our ancestors ate—yet just the idea of the Paleo Diet is challenged by many. This diet is based on the likelihood that millions of years of evolution of our nutritional requirements, as well as our ability to utilize certain foods and not others, should be taken into consideration in the modern diet. An animal requires certain nutrients to survive, and over tens of thousands or hundreds of thousands of years, it has developed the digestive system to absorb them.

For humans, when a new food or, even worse, a processed or genetically altered food is introduced, it may take thousands of years to re-evolve our systems to survive on it. The introduction of wheat—which became a staple when humans began farming it in large quantities thousands of years ago—made humans very unhealthy. Mummies of Egyptian farmers, who lived mostly on wheat, demonstrate evidence of many more diseases (such as crippling arthritis) than do mummies of the hunters and gatherers of the time, who had a simpler diet. The consumption of wheat products continues to make humans unhealthy today.

Now bring in the need for profit. Keeping food from spoiling by adding chemicals—sometimes poisons—or by genetically altering it can—and does—create harmful results.

Anyone really committed to the Paleo Diet can tell you that they know when they've eaten something processed; it's not pleasant. This was written about in the late 1930s in the Price-Pottenger studies of the introduction of "foods of commerce" to natives. At first they were made sick by the processed food, but within a few weeks, they were addicted to it.

In this book, I will attempt to clarify many misconceptions that have interfered with our ability to achieve optimal health, overcome or prevent disease, and slow down the aging process. In addition, I hope to give the reader the ability to know when a doctor is just treating symptoms versus working on an answer to what is causing the symptoms.

I also greatly hope that, somehow, I can bring to the reader the important role he or she plays in achieving a symptom-free life—one that has Great-Grandma or Great-Grandpa playing with the children and enjoying the fruits of his or her productive life—and not from a bed!

What You'll Find in this Book

This book lays out the severe dysfunction I see existing in our present-day approach to health—and what you can do about it. Each chapter contains an important principle about our health problems and how to shift the current medical paradigm. Here are the topics we're going to explore:

In chapter 1, "Left-Brained versus Right-Brained Thinking," we will look at one of the main reasons for the dysfunction in our medical system: the imbalance of left- and right-brained thinking. I believe that we need both, in order to succeed at understanding and achieving true health.

Chapter 2, "The Illusion of Treating Symptoms Only," looks at how the dysfunction manifests—primarily in the treatment of symptoms rather than the real cause of disease. While it always feels great for symptoms to be alleviated, many don't realize that if the cause is not treated, there will likely be other problems down the road. Such later problems will reduce the quality of life or require another drug to treat the symptoms caused by the side effects of the first one.

In my practice, I have had profound results using change in diet to alleviate symptoms and help patients restore their good health. In chapter 3, "Diet and Nutrition: Why They Matter," we'll talk about the difference between diet and nutrition, as well as the dangerous consequences of continuing to ignore the relationship between diet and disease.

Chapter 4, "The Danger of Food Allergies," extends this conversation to the serious consequences of food allergies and why it's critical for us to pay attention and do whatever is possible to correct these. In this chapter, we'll look at the "big eight" food allergies and symptoms that can arise when we fail to realize how certain foods may be harming us. We will also talk about the relationship of diet to telomeres, a part of our cells directly related to aging.

Chapter 5, "Fighting Inflammation with Diet," looks at one of the fundamental causes of many diseases. In this chapter, we'll talk specifically about which foods cause inflammation and which ones are high in anti-inflammatory properties.

Chapter 6 tackles the serious problem of the "Poisons in Processed Foods." We'll explore some of the things permitted in the United States that are banned in other countries. We'll also look at the pros and strengths of my diet of choice, the Paleo Diet.

In chapter 7, "The Importance of Supplementing Your Diet," we'll look at why it's essential to supplement—and the FDA's attitude toward supplementation.

"Legal Drug Abuse" is the topic of chapter 8. Here, I'll emphasize the importance of carefully reading about any prescription given to you by your doctor, the problem of side effects, the shortcomings of our thinking process when it comes to treating symptoms with medications—and the potential dangers.

In chapter 9, "Acupuncture: The Rise of Complementary and Alternative Medicine," I will share with you what I've learned about acupuncture as an alternative to anesthesia for surgery. This chapter includes an interview with the "Father of American Cardiology," Dr. Paul Dudley White. We'll look at this ancient healing art and the failure of the medical industry even to consider this and other successful therapies in lieu of or in addition to conventional medicine.

Chapter 10 is "Epidemiology: A Proposal to Save Billions and End Suffering." It explores the

field of epidemiology, the study of disease distribution in populations, and the lack of use of what
could be a profoundly important tool for us in
discovering the cause of disease in certain areas
or conditions.

This is followed by chapter 11, "Why Do We
Have to Fight the Government?" This book is
my contribution to standing up for what I see as
demagogy in our society.

Finally, chapter 12 answers the question,
"What Can YOU Do to Help?" This chapter em-
phasizes one of the main messages of this book,
that each of us must take responsibility for our
own health.

Let's get started!

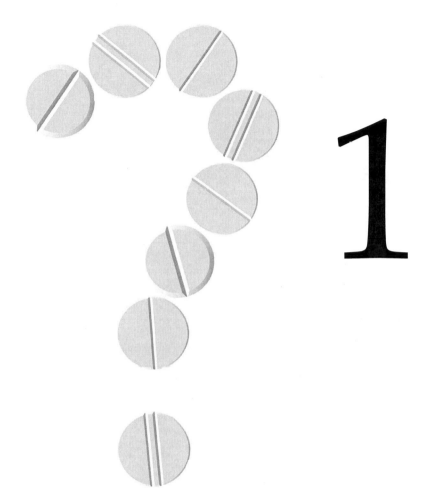

1

Left-Brained versus
Right-Brained Thinking

Left-Brained versus Right-Brained Thinking

Einstein once said that imagination is more important than knowledge. In other words, both a left-brained and a right-brained approach to life makes for a more holistic way to evaluate, make decisions, and live well. Knowledge, discipline, and memorization are left-brain activities; imagination and creativity are right-brain functions. Doctors and patients need to embrace both if we're going to have any chance at succeeding in creating a healthy society.

It's easy to get out of balance in favor of one kind of brain activity over the other. For example, we have sometimes seen entire societies succeed by taking another culture's invention and then, due to their superior discipline, mass-produce this product more efficiently than did the culture that invented the product. Japan and China have built their wealth this way in recent years. Yet in doing so, they've sacrificed creative development, often having to infiltrate our industry and patent offices to get new ideas.

You might ask why. Many years ago, a group of psychiatrists studying in Japan found that Japanese children were far more disciplined at earlier ages than were children in other countries. From young childhood, the children went on to disciplined schooling and then very defined careers. Throughout their education, learning involved strict memorization; not only was use of the right brain not encouraged, it wasn't even allowed to develop.

For some reason, the educational system in the United States has adopted many of Japan's approaches. This has developed in such a way that a right-brain-dominant child is often considered ADD or ADHD and given drugs, rather than having his or her right-brain strengths stimulated. In most colleges, the higher the education, the more left-brain-dominant the student becomes.

This would help explain why so many famous and successful people did not go to or finish college; they got out before their right brain was inactivated. The founders of Apple and Microsoft are good examples of this.

I experienced both left- and right-brain approaches at college. The worst instructor I had at Cal was a French literature professor. You had to interpret the books to his conclusions and philosophies—or you flunked. Needless to say, I received the worst grade ever in that course.

The best instructor I ever had was my calculus professor. He loved his work so much that he would get tears in his eyes describing what a formula meant. Integral calculus is a right-brain subject, far too vast for the left brain to conceive of. I was so turned on that I would save that homework for last, because it would overcome sleepiness. That course was my highest college achievement.

This is not to say that memorization is not essential to knowledge, but it is vital to understand that many of the subjects we're required to memorize may be found invalid in the future. If we lock onto the things we're forced to memorize and don't allow our right brain to challenge them, progress can't happen. Think where science would be if the student never challenged what he was taught. Yet look at the price a student might pay for challenging a professor or teacher in school.

Hanging onto the British system of measurement—inches, feet, pounds, ounces, and British Thermal Units (BTUs)—instead of the globally used metric system is absurd. Yet students are still forced to memorize many useless principles because someone or some group won't let go.

In medicine, the standard of care for cancer is unwavering, yet it's obsolete and has been for years. To make it worse, if a doctor tries something outside the "standard of care," even though it has been proven to work, he will almost always lose in our legal system if the treatment doesn't succeed. And "standard of care" can vary from state to state. Currently, for example, medical procedures are done quite successfully in Nevada that would not be allowed in California.

The persons making these rules are like the old guys that still wanted to use horses in World War II.

If you Google the names of some of history's "nonstandard of care" heroes—like Dr. Frank Shallenberger in Nevada or Dr. Stanislaw Burzynski in Texas, the ones that are willing to take chances—you'll find all kinds of negative information in the form of judgments and complaints. These are usually the opinions of another professional who disagrees with the practice because it is not the "standard of care" or "evidence based."

That does not imply that there are not bad alternative practitioners, who are there only to take advantage of the desperation one has when faced with a disease that appears fatal. Unfortunately, there are those without conscience who will do anything for money. On the other hand, the same thing is happening with our FDA—only the money comes from the drug companies. The movie *Burzynski* will open your eyes to the criminal activity going on within the institutions that are supposed to be protecting us.

I am not diverging from the subject that began this book. Many of these people are "well educated," or rather well-memorized, in medicine and pharmacology, which gives them a false sense of authority. And due to their lack of right-brain activity, they are almost totally unable to conceive of alternative ideas. One of the characteristics of left-brain-dominant people is that they become authoritative and opinionated, seeking positions as politicians, teachers, professors, and bureaucrats so that they can demonstrate their mastery of old information. Sadly, such people also seek positions in the medical field.

The only truly right-brained professors I have found in medicine are those who are there because they love the profession. They are not there to prove themselves. And the same thing is true in private practice: the best doctors are the ones who love what they do and crave further knowledge, realizing how much more there is yet to learn. As Werner Erhard related to me, the more intelligent minds know there is a lot they don't know, and the really intelligent realize they don't even know what they don't know.

One might think that someone associated with a college or right out of medical school with the latest knowledge would be the best doctor to go to. For the moment, he or she might be the best, but as unique circumstances pop up requiring a new approach, without the right brain heavily involved, such a person could be among the least qualified.

A very simple example from my own life—for which I thank my right brain—is the way I sew up a wound. Every medical student is taught to cleanse the area, then inject a numbing agent so that we can stitch without pain. But when I see a wound, I see a big hole. Why do I need to add more pain by making several more little holes? I merely spray the numbing agent into the wound along the edges, wait a little longer, and then stitch. If the patient still feels pain in a particular spot, a small injection from the wound side, which is already numb, will do the job. I also use a much thinner needle than most.

What it all boils down to is that the most important question a doctor can ask himself about a patient's medical problem is why? I don't care if it's just a bad complexion being seen by a dermatologist. Don't give the patient a drug, which has side effects and only covers the symptom. Ask, why does this patient have this problem?

In finding out what's causing acne, a doctor might prevent many future problems located in other areas of the body. Even though I'm not a dermatologist, for example, I have relieved my orthodontic patients of this horrible condition by having them simply eliminate dairy products from their diet.

Recently, I was with friends at an Italian restaurant when I saw someone I hadn't seen in months. He had really changed. I went over to talk to him and learned that he was being treated for pancreatic cancer at one of the top institutions in the world. Poor guy, he had recently retired and built his dream home.

I saw that he had just finished a large serving of angel hair pasta, so I asked if the doctors had brought up the relationship between cancer and diet. I knew what the answer would be. If he had been treated by one of those "illegal clinics" that I am familiar with— there would have been a multiple approach—including attention to diet, oxygen, and blood alkalinity. That plate of pasta is way up there on the Inflammatory Index—and inflammation is known to be the major cause of cancer (more on this in chapter 5).

I agreed to meet with my friend and supply him with references that would help him understand what he could do to have a chance at survival.

It is hard to understand why most physicians refuse to step outside the box of their traditional learning, ignoring unconventional or "alternative" approaches that could save lives. Yet we can't condemn physicians for refusing to step outside the box, since the educational system locked them in the box in the first place! This is not funny—it's real—and the system must be changed if we want the most from it.

It's not that the left-brain-dominant doctor is not compassionate—it's just that he or she has been taught that alternative medicine is bad, and that's that. What we need is a balanced approach.

Let me share another example from my own life. In 1970 I had been in an orthodontic practice for six years. It was quite apparent that the drug situation was out of control, and I began counseling teens, often ending up with over 100 teens meeting at my house because they just wanted to be acknowledged. This was a time when, if you weren't good-looking, a jock, or a cheerleader, you were no one.

I was overwhelmed with the work, so I got other adults to help out. Seeing that there was little or no communication going on between parents and teens, I proposed a center where kids and adults could go for help.

For over a year, I led this group—but we didn't seem to make any progress. I was a good leader (a right-brain quality) but not a good organizer and bookkeeper (left-brain abilities). So I brought in some men and women who were very successful at business—and the project took off.

Over forty years later, the Discovery Center is the most successful enterprise of its kind, with the community strongly behind it and a thrift shop that has raised over six million dollars. It has helped thousands of families and individuals through hard times, offering emotional help at whatever price they could afford. Being mostly right-brain-dominant, I could not have done this by myself.

It has since become clear to me that we need both right- and left-brain-dominant people to complement one another, not just in a project like the center, but in other areas of life as well.

In terms of medicine, thankfully, the movement in this country toward integrative medicine is gaining momentum. I'm grateful to be part of it.

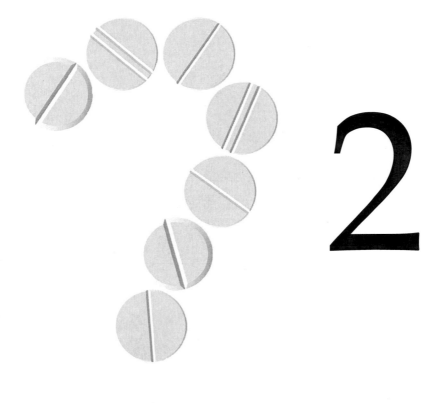

2

The Illusion of Treating Symptoms Only

The Illusion of Treating Symptoms Only

One of the most important ways to lead a symptom-free life is to understand that we can't just treat symptoms! Today's common practice of treating symptoms only can postpone an accurate diagnosis, even resulting in a possibly curable disease becoming fatal.

Let's take a rather common symptom that many people ignore and doctors give pills for: edema, which is unexplained swelling, usually in the lower legs. Oftentimes, if you look careful-ly, swelling can be seen in other areas as well—in the eyes, face, abdomen, and fingers.

It is extremely important to find out the cause of the edema—the *why*—as the answer could totally change your life for the better (in other words, don't give in and take something like a medication just to hide an illness). However, the usual practice for edema is to give a diuretic drug (i.e., Lasix or Diuril) that stimulates urination to take away the water causing the swelling.

In this treatment, there is no diagnosis of the underlying cause as to why water is causing the swelling, but the symptom goes away and everyone is happy. The patient is happy because his or her symptom is gone, the doctor is happy because he or she has done his job, and the insurance company is happy because the "cure" was so simple.

What really *should* happen is quite the opposite. The patient should demand to know why, and if lucky enough to have the perfect doctor, the patient will be thankful that he or she has a symptom that has caused either a simple problem (one that is easily cured) or a life-threatening illness to be properly examined and diagnosed.

Let's look at just a few of the possible causes of edema; there are many, and I'll discuss each one to show you why it's so important to go deeper to find the cause of the symptom. Caught early, these problems can be corrected; optimal health is possible. But it takes commitment.

Possible causes of edema include the following:

- Decreased albumin
- Improper sodium-to-potassium ratio
- Hormone imbalance
- Mitochondrial insufficiency
- Drugs

Let's look at each of these. **Albumin** is the major blood protein. It is made in the liver, and one of its functions is to prevent water from pooling in the tissues. Liver disease is a major cause of low albumin and can be due to excessive alcohol and fructose consumption. Several other liver problems can result from albumin deficiency, including cancer.

Kidney disease can also cause low albumin. So can a bad diet, low in protein, which can lead to bowel diseases, such as Crohn's disease or celiac disease. These, by the way, are actually misnamed as diseases; they are really symptoms of an underlying immune system problem, such as a food allergy. Again, the medical profession wants to treat the symptom instead of taking time to find the cause. I dropped twenty pounds in three weeks when I stopped eating gluten.

Excessive **salt** consumption is probably blamed the most for edema. What is left out in this reasoning is that the body must maintain an alkalinity similar to that of sea water—so the body will hang on to anything salty it can get to do so. You could be deficient in potassium, magnesium, or many other minerals. Supplementing to bring the right mineral balance can not only cure the edema, but it can also save you from problems associated with mineral deficiencies. Yet what are you told? Lower your salt consumption!

In some cases, that would be a good thing. It is always bad to eat excessive amounts of salt, especially in processed foods. Your body must get rid of the excess, unless you're very athletic and sweat a lot, in which case you might even need salt pills.

But another factor should be considered: water consumption. One cannot sweat or urinate without losing sodium, as well as other minerals. So increasing the amount of water you drink plus cutting down on the many forms of sodium salts you use (e.g. soy sauce, MSG, bicarbonate of soda, and processed foods) and adding potassium and magnesium supplements is a much more effective and healthy way to go.

Hormone imbalance can cause edema or water retention. In women, the progesterone to estradiol ratio can be the problem. Again, we need to look at the liver, for it is one of the factors controlling the balance of these hormones. Another big factor can be a diet low in vegetables, fruits, and berries. Too much coffee and alcohol can greatly affect the liver's function, as well.

As one reaches forty to fifty years of age, both men and women can greatly benefit from a detailed study of their hormones. Water retention is just one of many problems that can easily be corrected by a well-informed doctor or hormone specialist. One hormone, estradiol, can become elevated in men as well as women, because after fifty, some men convert testosterone into estradiol—a process that can be exacerbated by excessive alcohol intake. Too much estradiol (one of the estrogens) can lead to prostate cancer and heart disease, as well as to emotional and sexual problems.

Another hormone that should be checked in the case of edema is thyroid hormone. Low thyroid hormone can cause edema, but it can easily be controlled with replacement thyroid-hormone supplements.

Mitochondrial fitness could be the most important contributor to your health. Thousands of intracellular "bubbles" called mitochondria exist inside your cells to produce energy. Lack of these little guys can result in accelerated aging. Over half of the energy they produce is used just to push the sodium out of the cell to prevent water retention.

If you have water retention and you avoid

exercise, the chances are you have a condition of mitochondrial unfitness. Exercise is of extreme importance, not just to your heart but to the cells throughout your body.

Drugs and their side effects can cause major edema. Blood pressure drugs are among the biggest offenders, although there are many others that also produce edema. If you are prescribed a medicine, it's always good to go to your computer and look it up. Check the side effects, and be aware during the first six months of taking the drug of whether you are having any of the side effects. If so, your doctor should be informed and should possibly change the medication.

• • •

The five medical conditions we just went over are just a subset of those that could cause water retention. Yet they often are not even considered before a doctor prescribes a drug. What is important is that your body is telling you that there may be a disease that needs to be diagnosed and treated. Cancer, heart disease, congestive heart failure, liver, and kidney disease are among the most critical. When you have a symptom like edema, your doctor should order lab work, including a (complete blood count), a chemistry panel, and an electrolyte study. A C-reactive protein test is also a good idea.

After eliminating the life-threatening diseases, and before going to drugs to address only the symptom, diagnosis of non-life-threatening conditions such as the five discussed above should be pursued.

Eventually, even though many of these conditions are not really serious, as you grow older, your quality of life can be severely reduced and result in you spending your later years in assisted living, instead of at home enjoying happy activities with your family.

As for those impatient individuals who seek instant gratification and instant relief of symptoms, there are plenty of them. Their attitude is: Who cares about the future? Give me the pill. Many patients live by the rule, If it tastes good, eat it. This goes along with a sick toast I heard years ago: "Here's to hell; may the stay there be as pleasant as the way there."

Well, you don't have to wait for hell. You'll have plenty of pain and misery before you get there if you choose to live by rules like these.

I have to work hard to hold back my emotions with this type of patient. I will later pity them when they declare that they wish they had listened to those who wanted to help. Too many times, I have witnessed a friend or relative dying of lung cancer saying they wished they had listened to me. This is not the reward I would ever want—their realizing I was right and they were wrong.

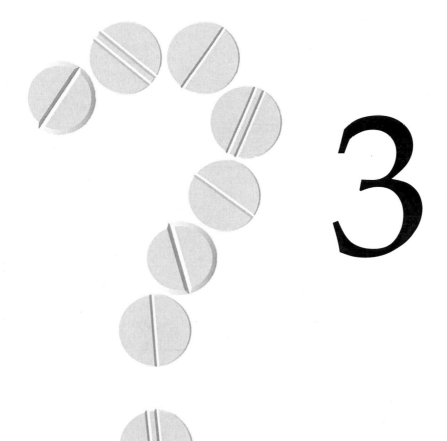

3

Diet and Nutrition:
Why They Matter

Diet and Nutrition: Why They Matter

For more than twenty-five years, I've been part of a Harvard research project linking eating and supplement habits to disease. During this time, I've learned a lot about relating these habits to the medical conditions one experiences throughout one's life. But how does the medical profession in general view diet and nutrition? In many cases, doctors deny there is any connection between diet and the diseases in their speciality.

Again, the big *why?* I have never had a doctor ask me to fill out anything about what I eat as part of my medical history. If I were a fast-food junkie—eating everything processed along with my soft drinks, beer, or wine—my health would be vastly different from that of a health-conscious person who eats a primarily vegetarian diet. Yet information that could be vital in diagnosing one's ill health is consistently overlooked or ignored.

In the case of some diseases, your eating and drinking habits are, without a doubt, the most important single factor. Yet how many people know that arthritis, an almost universal malady of the elderly, can be controlled by diet?

The following statement was given by a patient in Dr. Colin J. Dong's book, *New Hope for the Arthritic*:

About two-and-a-half years ago, a month after the birth of my child, I found myself extremely fatigued. I began to feel stiffness and pain in my joints, especially in the morning. At first I thought it was simply the aftereffects of my pregnancy. However, soon my joints started to swell—first in my fingers, then my wrists and shoulders, and finally down to my knees.

After completing a series of laboratory tests and x-ray examinations, the doctors told me that the laboratory tests showed I had rheumatoid arthritis. I was seriously ill for a whole year. I could not bathe myself, or dress myself, or hold my new baby; I could hardly walk.

I was taking 20 aspirins a day, and also, subsequently, cortisone, Indocid, and Butazolidin alka by mouth. The medicine also made me very ill. I had been taking gold shots too. But nothing seemed to help me, and I got worse and worse. Both of my knees became terribly inflamed and swollen. They became about twice the size of normal knees, and naturally I could not walk at all then.

The rheumatologist said that if I did not get better I would have to have them drained. That was what I should expect from the disease rheumatoid arthritis. The doctor made an appointment for me with the hospital to have the knees drained in two weeks.

In the meantime, I found The Arthritic's Cookbook. *I went on the diet. When I went back to the rheumatologist in two weeks, my knees were back down to normal size. He could not believe this at all. He said that he had not seen anything like this in his life.*

I do not take any more aspirin. I do not take anything now but a Naproxen and one Prednisone a day.

I do not have any pains anymore, and just a little stiffness once in a while. I'm not tired anymore during the day like I used to be.

I wonder if the rheumatologist ever asked what this patient ate, and if she happened to tell him, whether he looked into her diet. When I cured my daughter of asthma, the pediatric allergist never asked me what I did. I've noticed that without a balance of left brain and right brain, left-brain-dominant people typically don't question their own knowledge. Thinking "outside the box" is a right-brain phenomenon, essential for questioning one's self.

I can't think of any disease or medical problem that cannot be prevented or at least helped by changing one's diet. Dr. Otto Warburg, in 1925, announced he had discovered a major cause and possible cure for cancer. He received the Nobel Prize for this in 1931. The cause: low blood oxygen and high blood acidity. Both these factors can be corrected, either partially or totally, by diet and nutrition.

By the way, eighty-three years later, treatments using this discovery are not yet considered "evidence based" or "standard of care."

Diet versus Nutrition: What's the Difference?

Diet refers to the foods you eat. Nutrition has more to do with what actually is assimilated from the food into the blood and lymphatic system. This can be altered by our body's ability to process what it is given, and it requires a healthy stomach and intestine, necessary enzymes, and a healthy liver. Much of the time, because what we take in is inadequate in nutrients or not completely digested and assimilated, supplements may be necessary.

There is as much misinformation as there is information about diets. I have studied some anticancer diets that are so ridiculous it downright takes the joy out of not just eating, but out of life itself.

With the exception of someone who is already damaged by illness, there is growing evidence that a diet that stays as close to what humanity ate while evolving is what we should try to achieve. Some call it the Caveman Diet, but most refer to it as the Paleo Diet. Processed foods are out. Fast foods are out. Alcohol is greatly reduced, as are carbohydrates and sugar. Saturated fats are avoided, as are vegetable oils. Genetically altered foods are out. Proper food combining is *in*. Proper herbs and supplements are *in*.

As one might expect, critics of the Paleo Diet are numerous. The following, taken from Wikipedia, is an example of how critics consider themselves "experts" and feel qualified to condemn this diet:

A 2011 ranking by *U.S. News & World Report,* involving a panel of 22 experts, ranked the Paleo diet lowest of the 20 diets evaluated based on factors including health, weight-loss, and ease of following. These results were repeated in the 2012 survey, in which the diet tied with the Dukan diet for the lowest ranking out of 25 diets; *U.S. News & World Report,* stated that their experts "took issue with the diet on every measure." However, one expert involved in the ranking stated that a "true Paleo diet might be a great option: very lean, pure meats, lots of wild plants. The modern approximations . . . are far from it." He added that "duplicating such a regimen in modern times would be difficult."

Notice that one of the criteria used to rank this diet in this report was "ease of following." These "experts" were clearly demonstrating their lack of expertise. Yes, this diet is much harder to follow than grabbing a Big Mac or deli sandwich. But I have been on this diet for years and find it quite easy to follow.

I speculate that these "experts" might regard the Paleo Diet as hard to follow   because after being on the diet for a while, if they eat processed foods, they get a sick feeling—sometimes becoming quite sick.

There is no question that a commitment to optimal health takes a lot of effort. But the rewards make it well worth it.

Wikipedia goes into great detail regarding the Paleo Diet. I found one section of the research there to be very important and worthy of including here:

> Since the end of the Paleolithic period, several foods that humans rarely or never consumed during previous stages of their evolution have been introduced as staples in their diet. With the advent of agriculture and the beginning of animal domestication roughly 10,000 years ago, during the Neolithic Revolution, humans started consuming large amounts of dairy products, beans, cereals, alcohol, and salt. In the late eighteenth and early nineteenth centuries, the

Industrial Revolution led to the large-scale development of mechanized food-processing techniques and intensive livestock farming methods that enabled the production of refined cereals, refined sugars, and refined vegetable oils, as well as fattier domestic meats, which have become major components of Western diets.

Such food staples have fundamentally altered several key nutritional characteristics of the human diet since the Paleolithic era, including glycemic load, fatty acid composition, macronutrient composition, micronutrient density, acid-base balance, sodium-potassium ratio, and fiber content.

These dietary compositional changes have been theorized as risk factors in the pathogenesis of many of the so-called "diseases of civilization" and other chronic illnesses that are widely prevalent in Western societies, including obesity, cardiovascular disease, high blood pressure, type 2 diabetes, osteoporosis, autoimmune diseases, colorectal cancer, myopia, acne, depression, and diseases related to vitamin and mineral deficiencies.

What this report indicates is that over millions of years, the human has developed a digestive system than can become quite ill if it is forced to eat only recently developed foods that weren't available when human bodies were first developing. It's quite logical: it's like putting gasoline in a diesel engine—only worse.

In my practice, I have found that acne can be caused by milk, which is rather new to our diets. Psoriasis and many other skin problems can be caused by gluten, which can also be responsible for celiac disease. Again, grains, to the extent we eat them, are quite recent factors in our digestive evolution.

Why Proper Digestion Is So Important

Earlier, I mentioned that diet is what we eat and nutrition is the result of what nutrients actually get into our blood and lymphatic system. Even if your diet is close to perfect, it must be properly digested, with the nutrients broken down, allowing proper conversion into substances that can enter the blood and lymphatic system. It starts in the mouth, where even at the beginning of the digestive process, there can be deficiencies or diseases causing improper digestion and malnutrition. This is treated by the field of medicine called gastroenterology.

Again, there are those in this field who treat just the symptoms. So let's look at what proper digestion involves. The process of digestion is quite complex, and rather than go into extensive details of the process, it is my desire to point out things that can go wrong due to factors that can often be controlled or changed, simply by altering our lifestyle, habits, and activities.

Beginning at the starting point of digestion, the mouth, it helps to have the ability to chew one's food and mix it with the first digestive enzymes that come into play, which break down starch and fat. A healthy mouth gets this started, but having numerous missing teeth may cause food to have no contact with these parts of the mouth, preventing ideal digestion from happening.

Next, the food enters the stomach, where there may be more problems. The simplest problem occurs as a result of improper food combining. For example, meat and potatoes have opposite digestive needs; protein requires acidic processing, and starch requires alkaline processing. The digestion becomes less efficient, therefore, when one improperly combines the two, and this can result in incomplete digestion and a loss of energy.

The same thing can happen with bread and meat. That sandwich at lunch can mean a sleepy afternoon. A salad or meat with a vegetable works much better. But what do so many people do? They take an energy drink or drink coffee all afternoon to make up for the effects of improper food combining. They might even require an antacid, which further interferes with digestion.

One of the common problems in this area is *acid reflux*, medically called *gastroesophageal reflux disease* (GERD). With heavily advertised over-the-counter remedies, such as Prilosec, GERD is handled well, and now doctors are not the only ones treating symptoms—we are.

Untreated GERD can lead to many complications, including cancer. It is one of many stomach problems called diseases, which are actually symptoms that need to be properly diagnosed in order to correct them.

Let's continue with a brief description of the remaining process. In the stomach, very large carbohydrate, fat, and protein molecules are broken down into a liquid called chyme. This liquid enters the duodenum and goes on to the small intestine to be mixed, forming a more basic chemical structure that can be absorbed through the walls of the stomach and the small and large intestines. The liver, pancreas, and glands of the intestinal walls all secrete products that break our food down into chyme, but they can only provide them to the extent that these organs are healthy and not abused.

All of the functions are controlled by a complex system of hormones that control the enzyme production and nerves that control the muscular activity that moves the products of the food along. This nervous system is known as the autonomic nervous system, because we don't control it, although we can strongly influence it.

The autonomic system is made up of the sympathetic and parasympathetic nervous systems. If you're stressed, the sympathetic nervous system causes the release of adrenaline, which slows or stops the muscles causing that sick feeling that comes along with stress and distress. Again, drugs can be used to cover the symptoms of stress, but wouldn't it be nice if you could change your lifestyle to eliminate stress and avoid the serious side effects associated with these types of drugs?

By the time the digested product reaches the colon, or large intestine, almost all the nutrients are absorbed. Water, minerals, and vitamins are absorbed in the colon, and biotin, as well as vitamin K, is produced there. A low-fiber diet, as well as antibiotic use, can greatly affect the efficiency of the colon, and so can parasites and foreign bacteria.

Bacteria are extremely important to digestion. In fact, our emphasis on cleanliness and avoidance of non-pasteurized foods requires supplementing our diets with probiotics to give us the badly needed bacteria stripped by the process of pasteurization. Organic beer and wine also contain nutrients that are lost when pasteurization is done.

How does alcohol figure into this discussion? When one combines a low-fiber diet with heavy bourbon or Scotch consumption, the tar products caused by charcoal filtering in the process of making whiskey can be deposited in the *diverticuli,* or small folds of the wall of the colon, leading to colon cancer. High-fiber diets tend to cleanse the colon, helping to prevent the folds of the colon from collecting debris; it's believed that the major cause of diverticulitis is a low-fiber diet. Once these "pouches" form, debris tends to be caught up and held there, potentially causing irritation. This disease is quite painful—but it can be prevented.

Having a little more understanding of the digestive system may lead you to wonder about the disease called Crohn's disease. This is the name medicine has given to an irritated colon. And the typical attitude toward it is this: Oh, now that we call it a disease, let's give it a drug like Prednisone (a steroid with multiple side effects, some of which are quite dangerous).

BUT WAIT! THIS IS NOT A DISEASE, IT IS A SYMPTOM—and it needs diagnosis. *Why* is the colon irritated?

I had an eight-year-old girl in my practice being treated with Prednisone for Crohn's disease. Her face looked like a little pumpkin, it was so swollen from the side effects. I referred her to a holistic doctor, and the cause was discovered to be sensitivity to wheat and dairy. Because of the damage to her colon and immune system, it required over six months of supplementation to re-establish her health, regain her pretty face, and allow her to go on with a normal life. In this case, researching the *why* resulted in finding the true disease—a food sensitivity—and finding a simple cure: not eating those foods to which she was sensitive.

In studying acupuncture, I found a correlation between Crohn's disease and migraine headaches. The meridian associated with the colon begins just ahead of the acromion (a little bump on the scapula next to the arm). This is referred to as C1. A meridian that travels up the side of the head crosses C1 at that point. In my temporomandibular joint dysfunction (TMJ) practice, when the patient complains of migraines, I touch the spot where it hurts and sometimes feel an electric-like impulse. When a chilling agent (ethyl chloride) is sprayed there, the headache miraculously disappears. How many Western-trained physicians would more likely laugh at this rather than try to understand *why* this works?

The use of antibiotics can disturb the normal intestinal flora, thus causing digestive problems and discomfort. A holistic approach to correct this is detoxification and administration of pro-biotics to re-establish the proper flora.

It's all quite logical when you look at our health holistically. We have an incredible, wonderful gift—our body—that deserves to be treasured and nurtured—not abused, either by ourselves or practitioners. The rewards are well worth the effort.

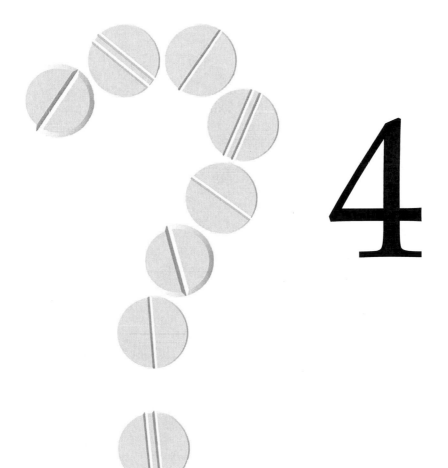

4

The Danger of Food Allergies

The Danger of
Food Allergies

Let's now extend the topic of diet and nutrition to a serious and common problem suffered by so many: food allergies. Common food allergies normally just cause discomfort, skin problems, and lack of joy in life. But some allergies can be fatal. Let's take a closer look at allergies and how we might treat them more effectively through changes in diet than by using some of the more conventional methods.

The Big Eight

Food allergies can result in a host of uncomfortable symptoms. So if you are sensitive or allergic to any food, it's important to know and avoid that food. Eating any food that you're allergic to increases adrenaline and cortisol, which are damaging chemicals in the body, and it can make life really miserable. And life is stressful enough without throwing a little more adrenaline into the mix when we eat.

The most common food allergens for humans are referred to as "the big eight": milk, eggs, peanuts, tree nuts, seafood, shellfish, soy, and wheat. To not avoid such foods when you're sensitive to them is like begging nature to make you sick more often, saying: "Please bring on skin problems, please congest my nose, and let me sneeze my head off during allergy season." Even worse, you're also begging nature to age you faster and make you less attractive.

Food allergies can manifest in a number of ways:

- Skin conditions—eczema, psoriasis, hives, acne, and canker sores
- Nasal congestion and sinusitis—forces one to breathe through the mouth and snore (partial cause of sleep apnea)
- Angioedema—swelling of the lips, tongue, and general mucous membranes, sometimes making it hard to breathe
- Throat problems—difficulty swallowing and hoarse voice

- GI tract issues—gastric ulcer, gallbladder pain, bleeding, heartburn, abdominal pain, nausea, and vomiting
- Mental problems—depression, irritability, nervous and emotional instability, and abnormal tiredness
- Heart attacks (angina)
- Epilepsy
- Dizziness and fainting
- Anaphylactic shock (life-threatening)
- A feeling of discomfort, tiredness, and "yuckiness" in the stomach

There are several ways to test for food allergies, such as skin-sensitivity tests, blood tests, and others, but the most reliable method I've found is just eating certain foods you want to test and measuring your reaction to them.

There is also the Coca Pulse Test, introduced in 1956 by Dr. Arthur Coca. The method by which this test is done requires some effort, but it works. Because you do it yourself, it is by far the least expensive of any test I know.

This method was discovered when Dr. Coca was visiting his wife in the hospital. She had suffered several heart attacks, and the future was not looking good. It was just after dinner, and her pulse rate was extremely elevated. He noted what she had eaten for dinner (beef and potatoes) so he could test for possible correlations between her symptoms and food. After further testing, he found many foods that did not raise her heart rate, and limiting her diet to those foods, she lived a normal life.

Here's how Dr. Coca's test works. When one is exposed to an allergen, one of the body's first responses is the release of adrenaline. When adrenaline is released, heart rate increases. So you start the test by eating any food you want to test on day one, noticing if there's an increase in heart rate—which means you're likely allergic to that food.

But some foods are sneaky. If you haven't eaten the food being tested for some time, you might not get a reaction. So step two is to eat the same food four days later on an empty stomach. Our immune system has now had a chance to recognize that food. If you're allergic to it, your heart rate will go up again, and once again you may feel some discomfort. Eliminating that food from your diet will do wonders for your health. (If you are very allergic, this test will be conclusive, but when it is questionable, further testing is necessary.)

Although he was recognized throughout the world for his discovery and taught at Cornell, Heidelberg, the University of Pennsylvania, and Columbia, medical institutions would not accept Dr. Coca's findings. But his book is in the public domain and can be printed from the Internet. The following is a quote from the publisher of his book, Lyle Stuart:

This book is being published because the people who have been helped by the Coca technique convinced Dr. Coca that there was no need to wait half a century for the medical recognition which must eventually come.

We convinced him that by informing the layman, he would hasten the day when the medical profession would be forced to seriously examine these findings and his technique.

When that day comes, the physician will apply them too . . . and millions of men and women will be helped by Dr. Coca's important contribution to the health and well-being of mankind.

It has been much more than half a century, and that day is yet to come—although many open-minded doctors follow his work.

Luckily for my family, I carry the gene for allergies to wheat and milk. Why do I say we're lucky? Both those foods are undesirable if optimal health is desired. We are so brainwashed by the media that when I mention this, people think I'm nuts—even un-American!

Robert Cohen is the author of *Milk—The Deadly Poison*, a book that clearly proves milk is not for humans and can do great harm if consumed. I could write on and on about this subject, but even if you just look at it logically, it is unnatural to drink another animal's milk. Nowhere in nature does this occur, yet doctors readily recommend that we drink it for the calcium. Tell me, doctor, where does the cow get calcium? From vegetables!

As I brought up earlier, wheat is overrated in the Western diet, and recent findings reveal that as you age, if you want older, more wrinkled skin, whole wheat is the answer. Psoriasis and celiac disease, among many maladies, are also associated with wheat, mainly gluten (the protein in wheat). It contains other irritants as well.

Other Problems Associated with Food Allergies

An underlying problem associated with not correcting food allergies is that over time, regular stress, added to the damage done to the organ where the allergic reaction takes place, can lead to other problems that arise due to that organ's inability to function properly.

In the description of the digestive system in chapter 3, it was shown how the assimilation of the food we eat is dependent on organs releasing enzymes to break down that food. Enough abuse to an organ can actually cause that organ to develop an inability to break down the food, causing nutritional deficiencies in turn; the entire body suffers. Unfortunately, one of the problems of specialties in medicine is that one specialist can be treating a condition in the area of his specialty, not knowing it's being caused by a problem in the area of another specialist.

An example of such an occurrence might be a psychiatrist treating depression or anxiety caused by an enzyme deficiency or food allergy. The drugs used for these emotional problems work only on the symptom, and they can have severe side effects that will not stop returning, because the cause of the symptom is a nutritional problem, not a psychiatric one.

A dermatologist might be prescribing a steroid ointment for psoriasis when the problem is actually gluten sensitivity. The psoriasis is not going to go away until the cause is removed. Meanwhile, keep in mind that these steroids would not be obtainable by prescription only if there weren't problems that could occur with their use.

Other adverse responses to foods include food intolerance, toxin reactions, and pharmacological reactions. The true food allergy occurs as a reaction of the body to proteins that are not completely broken down by the digestive process into amino acids. The body mistakenly identifies these proteins as harmful and tags them with immunoglobulin E (IgE). Once tagged, these proteins are considered invaders, and the immune system sends in cells to attack, triggering an allergic reaction. This reaction can vary from dermatitis to respiratory distress to death resulting from anaphylaxis.

Even when death is not a threat, these other food intolerances must be dealt with, because damage to some part of our system may and does occur. With the exception of progressive inoculations of the allergen, meaning starting with minute doses and gradually building up the dose over months—which doesn't even always work—there is no cure except to avoid the food containing that protein.

One of the ways you can become allergic to a food, particularly one with an unusual protein, is to eat it frequently. This happened to me when I was an ocean diver—I ate so much abalone that I became allergic to it. In fact, I became allergic to crustaceans in general: crab, shrimp, and lobster. One year of *immunotherapy* (progressive injections) cured the latter allergies, but the treatment for abalone was so painful I had to stop it. So I stopped eating abalone, and today, I eat scallops—which are related to abalone—only about once a month.

One mistake I see in medicine is doctors telling someone he or she is allergic to shellfish, which typically includes crab, shrimp, lobster, clams, oysters, and more. But clams are about as distant in their evolution from crustaceans as humans are. I recommend that doctors take a little more time to find out *exactly* what the patient is allergic to—and that patients demand it! Each of these foods can be tested for.

Basically, the only treatments for food allergies are avoidance and immunotherapy desensitization through progressive dosage treatments over time. If one has a food allergy, there is always the chance that a severe reaction can occur. If this is true for you, it's recommended that you carry an injectable form of epinephrine (EpiPen). If you have ever had a severe reaction, you should wear a medical alert bracelet. And don't depend on asking a waiter if there is any form of peanut in the dish—ask the chef. I know of a local girl who died by not doing so.

Aside from the discomfort, possible danger, and inconvenience of food allergies, there is another very important reason to deal with them. Any time the functions of the body are interrupted, harmed, interfered with, or damaged, there is the potential for one of our systems not to function properly or even to stop functioning. Continued exposure to a protein that brings on an allergic reaction can keep putting stress on the glands that respond to allergens, such as the adrenal gland. Among the functions of this gland are the production of adrenaline and steroids. Just like you, our glands get tired when they're overworked and can't produce as efficiently.

Just this week, one of my patients who dropped dairy and gluten from her diet was able to discontinue using an inhaler for asthma. Her own system, no longer being abused by allergenic foods, can now handle the environmental problems causing her asthma.

Protecting our Wonderful Telomeres

Over the last couple of decades, the discovery of little things called telomeres has opened new fields of research. Telomeres occur on the tips of our genes and have a lot to do with the aging process and morbidity (occurrence of illness). Each time a cell divides, the telomeres in its genes become a little shorter and weaker. Once they're gone, life ends.

Excessive stress, as well as malnutrition, is one of many factors that accelerate the decay of telomeres. Once the body has been abused, something must be done to re-establish its health. Many institutions, including Harvard Medical School and the University of California, are looking into alternative medicine as a way to approach this problem.

I have seen herbal medicine work wonders in this area. In fact, Harvard has found that certain herbs can stimulate the production of telomerase, which is responsible for repairing telomeres—essentially reversing the aging process. The Nobel Prize in Physiology or Medicine was given to Elizabeth H. Blackburn, Carol W. Greider, and Jack W. Szostak in 2009 for this discovery.

Of course, it's good to remember that preventing the damage in the first place is so much easier. As we discussed in the previous chapter, no matter how good your diet is, your body only gets what you are capable of properly digesting. Most of us just aren't perfect, and we spend a little too much time abusing ourselves and then having to make up for it. Sometimes we think we can get away with abusing our body a little here and there. Then reality sets in, and we have to face up to it or suffer.

In chapter 7, I will address a few of the ways in which we can supplement our diet to repair some of the damage.

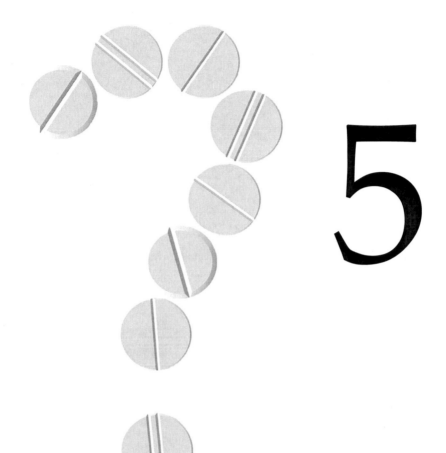

5

Fighting Inflammation with Diet

Fighting Inflammation
with Diet

L et's turn now to another major cause of discomfort and disease: inflammation. We've already talked about the high volume of misinformation about proper nutrition Western medicine feeds us—any consideration of foods that create an inflammatory response is largely ignored.

For example, as you are probably aware, the dietary guidelines issued by the U.S.Department of Agriculture (USDA) have been revised over time but continue to be inaccurate. Dairy, especially milk consumption, continues to be promoted. And the USDA continues to give cholesterol a bad rap.

Then, to top it off, the USDA's ChooseMyPlate guidelines recommend that adults get anywhere from six to eight servings of grains in their daily diet. These starches can be quite inflammatory, especially if you're sensitive to them—and a high percentage of people are. I would be miserable on this diet.

Rarely can you trust traditional Western doctors about what to eat. Doctors get very little training in nutrition, and apparently so do some nutritionists (judging by the website ChooseMyPlate.gov). Yet doctors consider themselves authorities, competent to give us advice on eating. Advice like this: diet has nothing to do with arthritis, you must drink milk for calcium, and you should use margarine instead of butter.

Far more important is to take a holistic approach and determine what your individual needs are. There is almost no "one diet fits all." It's best to educate yourself or seek the advice of a naturopath or holistic physician. We can also explore what foods create inflammation and which ones counter it.

What to Avoid

Let's begin with foods everyone should avoid. Keep in mind that some foods that create inflammation (except for the poisonous ones) can and should be consumed, but along with anti-inflammatory foods. Certain meats are moderately inflammatory, for example, but if you put meat on top of a large salad dressed with extra-virgin olive oil, the overall meal will fight inflammation, as well as give you some CoQ10 and many other nutrients.

Resources are available where you can look up the Inflammatory Index or Inflammatory Factor (IF) rating of a food. Once you look up a food, it tends to stick in your mind when you're planning your meals. Here's a list of strongly inflammatory foods that should always be avoided:

- **Sugar:** Since entering the field of dentistry, I have always wondered, if sugar rots your teeth, what else is it destroying? In nature, sweet foods are usually good for you, but man has learned to make the sweet flavor through different means. The sugar in a Coke equals ten sugar cubes. High-fructose corn syrup is doubly bad; you not only get the glycemic effects, but the fructose produces liver fat, creating cirrhosis.

- **Cooking Oils:** High omega-6 levels in vegetable oils promote inflammation. Corn oil gets deposited directly into the arterial wall once it's oxidized, causing atherosclerosis.

- **Polyunsaturated Vegetable Oils:** These oils—such as grape seed, cottonseed, safflower, corn, and sunflower oil—are all high in omega-6 and low in omega-3, and when used in cooking, they can easily become trans fats.

- **Trans Fats:** Fat is an essential factor in causing food to spoil. The food industry has found that by changing fats to trans fats through hydrogenation, the shelf life of a food can be increased. Partially hydrogenated oils, such as margarine and vegetable shortening, are inflammatory foods. Deep-fried foods are loaded with trans fats when cooked in vegetable oil. Cotton seed oil is already high on the Inflammatory Index, even before heating.

- **Commercially Raised Grain-Fed Meats:** Animals raised to produce these meats are fed a diet high in omega-6 fatty acids. Due to their cramped living conditions, they gain excess fat and contain high saturated fats. To make them grow faster, they're given hormones and antibiotics. An inflammatory food is the result.

- **Dairy Products:** Researchers have found that the ability to digest milk after infancy is abnormal. Milk is a common allergen that triggers the inflammatory process, resulting in gastric distress, rashes, acne, and respiratory problems such as asthma.

- **Red Meat and Processed Meat:** A chemical exists in some red meats called Neu5Gc. The body can produce an antibody to this molecule, which creates low-grade inflammation that persists for long periods of time. There is a high correlation between colon cancer and the consumption of red meats. Feed-lot grain feeding, including excessive grain feeding of chicken and turkeys, makes it even worse.

- **Refined Grains:** Over-refining of grains causes this food to become an inflammatory agent similar to sugar (a source of practically empty calories with a high glycemic index). Even whole grains can be responsible for celiac disease, and they have been found to be responsible for early aging of the skin.

Alcohol: Regular consumption can create inflammation in the esophagus, larynx, and liver. Small amounts can be tolerated, but heavy use is a killer.

Artificial Food Additives: Eating fresh is the answer. Processed foods contain flavor enhancers such as MSG, high-fructose corn syrup, and aspartame, as well as preservatives such as BHA and BHT. Corn syrup has been found to stimulate one's appetite, so our everloving bread producers are adding this nutrient to improve their financial health. MSG is a contributor to atherosclerosis.

Any Food You Are Sensitive To: If a food makes you feel uncomfortable, you should check into it. Some of the more common suspects are gluten, milk, eggs, legumes, and nightshade vegetables (eggplant, green peppers, and tomatoes). Medical tests are not always conclusive; home tests are available.

The majority of people I discuss the Paleo Diet with immediately say that it must really be difficult not only to follow, but also to cook. Well, that's true—if you call warming up something from the deli, frozen section, or processed food section "cooking." Foods that are freshly cooked under your supervision can be so much more nutritious and anti-inflammatory. Be careful not to overcook, as overcooking can severely deplete a food and sometimes even change it into an inflammatory food.

Fortunately for me, I have always enjoyed cooking. But even if you don't, once you grow accustomed to cooking Paleo, it's easy. And when you experience the great feelings of improved health, you will never want to go back.

As part of my diet, I occasionally reward myself with a homemade apple pie or some other great dessert—and I mean exceptional, since it's just once in a while. I will also go out for a steak or prime rib once a month. Interestingly, though, now that my health is the best it's ever been, my enthusiasm for the feel-good reward that used to be brought on by these splurges has decreased.

The Big Plus Foods

The discovery of the importance of controlling chronic inflammation has opened the doors to those who want to take a proactive part in preventing or even curing horrible diseases. To help you even further, the Inflammatory Index I mentioned above has been established for foods to help you tell the bad from the good when it comes to shopping for meals. Some important foods do fall a little on the inflammatory side, but understanding the index will let you know what to serve with that food or what to have at the next meal to balance it out.

The following is a list of some of the best anti-inflammatory foods one can eat:

- **Olive Oil (extra virgin):** This oil is so good for you that you can consider it a food supplement. Great for the skin too.

- **Organic Vegetables:** Especially broccoli, kale, brussels sprouts, and bok choy. All veggies are great, but these are especially anti-inflammatory.

- **Wild Salmon (not farmed).** This is a great source of omega-3 oil. On the Inflammatory Index, most fish score high for anti-inflammation. If you don't like fish, it may be the result of not knowing how to buy it or cook it. Overcooking can destroy flavor and make fish too dry. And sometimes what's being sold in the market isn't fresh. Being a fisherman, I can tell how fresh it is, and there are times I would throw some of it out. Find a salesperson you can rely on to tell you how fresh the fish is.

- **Garlic and Onions:** Garlic is very high on the anti-inflammatory index. An onion placed on a baking sheet with a little olive oil and cooked until tender is not only tasty but high on the anti-inflammatory index.

- **Ginger:** Contains many benefits in addition to being high on the index.

- **Sweet Potato:** So many good qualities, including fiber, beta-carotene, minerals, and vitamins.

- **Blueberries (organic only):** Organic because they are too small to allow for effective washing off of pesticides. These berries are so nutritious that they're almost like taking a drug for good health.

- **Turmeric:** Multiple benefits, in addition to being a tasty herb.

- **Papaya:** Loaded with vitamins plus a protein-digesting enzyme, papain, which improves digestion.

- **Shiitake Mushrooms:** Great eating, with anti-inflammatory properties as well as being a good source of vitamin D. Don't overcook or deep fry.

- **Green Tea:** Contains anti-inflammatory flavonoids, as well as antioxidants.

Finally, the information we need to take control of the quality of our lives is becoming available. With this knowledge, we can live a vital, youthful life that's much longer than average and have a lot more fun. If the doctor you go to doesn't agree with what you're learning here, find a doctor who does and is happy that you want to be part of what it takes to have the best health.

A couple of years ago, I came upon this true story in *The Huffington Post* from Dr. Mark Hyman, MD, about his Western medicine-treated patient:

> *Take, for example, a man who came to see me recently. He wanted to climb a mountain and asked for my help to get healthy. He was 57 years old and took about 15 medications for six different inflammatory conditions: high blood pressure, pre-diabetes, colitis, reflux, asthma, and an autoimmune disease of his hair follicles called alopecia.*
>
> *When I asked him how he felt, he said, "Great." I told him I was surprised because he was on so many medications.*
>
> *Yes, he said, but everything was very well controlled with the latest medications prescribed by the top specialists he saw in every field: the lung doctor for his asthma, the gastroenterologist for his colitis and reflux, the cardiologist for his high blood pressure, the endocrinologist*

for his pre-diabetes, the dermatologist for his hair loss.

But [I asked] did any of those specialists ask him why he had six different inflammatory diseases and why his immune system was so pissed off? Was it just bad luck that he "got" all these diseases—or was there something connecting all these problems?

He looked puzzled and said no.

I then searched for and uncovered the cause of his problems: gluten. He had celiac disease, an autoimmune disease related to eating gluten, the protein found in wheat, barley, rye, spelt, and oats.

Six months later he came back to see me. He had lost 25 pounds; no longer had high blood pressure, asthma, reflux, or colitis; and had normal bowel movements for the first time in his life. His hair was even growing back. And he was off nearly all his medications.

I just wish there were more doctors like Dr. Hyman. But even if you are lucky enough to have one like him, you still can't get out of your own responsibilities. You have to take part in your health.

This is not something to put off. You can look forward to an active, intelligent senior life. The "comfort food junkie" and "couch potato" will only be able to watch from their free scooters and beds with envy.

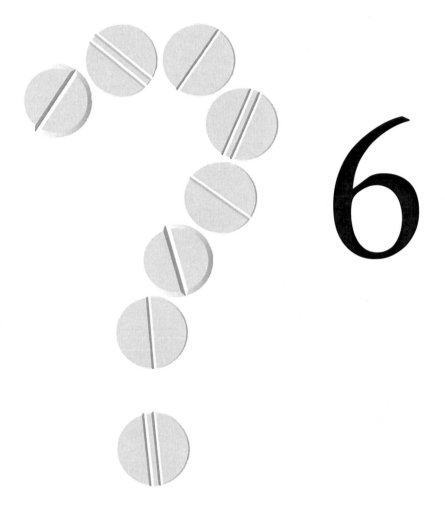

6

Poisons in Processed Foods

Poisons in Processed Foods

Now that we know how important it is to avoid substances that cause inflammation, let's look at one of the worst culprits: processed foods. They contain more than half of the inflammatory substances listed in the previous chapter—especially sugar and fat. And in order to turn your taste buds on, the food industry is not happy with just sugar and fat: they use high-fructose corn syrup and hydrogenated trans fats—which are even worse for your heart. In this case, the real motive is not just to preserve the food—it's greed (these products are cheaper).

Why are we not more informed about the poisons in these foods?

It has always bothered me that we go through twelve years of school without learning much at all about our bodies. It seems to me that our education should first include what makes up the complex structure we live in and how to take care of it. Unfortunately, the most important object you will ever own doesn't come with an operating manual. And for some reason, our society doesn't feel it is important enough to teach us about.

There should be a course in physiology from K through 12. I used to offer a class to fourth graders on what tobacco does to you—a course that included rather gross slides of cancer and post-surgical patients still smoking through a hole in their throat. I also showed them photos of the cancer caused by chewing tobacco, with testimonies from baseball players.

This was only one hour in one day of school. But these kids went home and raised hell with their parents who smoked. Can you imagine what could be done if every day there were a period dedicated to taking care of your body? It would mean billions less for the medical and pharmaceutical industries, not to mention the tobacco industry.

Part of the medical history that you fill out for your doctor should include the foods you eat: do you eat processed foods, do you read the labels, and how often do you eat these foods? Heart disease has been found to be much more serious when inflammation is present. And processed foods contribute greatly to inflammation—a major factor in heart disease.

So let's look more closely at this category of foods—how they contribute to our suffering and why we should avoid them.

What are Processed Foods— and What's the Big Deal?

Almost any food in a package, box, or can is processed. What does "processed" mean, and why is it done? Processed foods are real foods that have been altered in some way to enhance their flavor and shelf life and make them "safer." Such processing kills bacteria and other organisms that would spoil the food and not allow it to be shipped long distances or stored in markets.

Natural fats can quickly go rancid, for example, but when the natural fat in food is replaced with cheap trans fats, the food can last months. Adding chemicals, heating, irradiating, milling, and pressure treating are also used to extend shelf life and, in most cases, alter the food to be much less nutritious—even devoid of nutrition, in some cases.

I like to refer to these foods as empty calories. Empty calories do not supply the nutrients necessary for their digestion and assimilation, which prevents the body from getting some of its important vitamins and nutrients and which leaves the body depleted. White rice and alcohol are examples of empty calories, and they can cause loss of B-complex vitamins, damaging many organs, especially the liver. So you can see that, when processed, even potentially nutritious foods can be altered to become indirect poisons.

The following is a list of some of the chemicals added to processed foods and their effects on your health and well-being:

Chemical	Purpose	Possible Health Damage or Symptom	Usual Treatment
Canthaxanthin	Makes the meat of farmed salmon red	Retinal damage to the eye	Ophthalmology
MSG	Flavor enhancer	Headaches, chest pain, dizziness, mood swings	Pills
Propylene glycol	Emulsifier	Developmental/ reproductive issues, allergies, neurotoxicity, endocrine disruption	Misdiagnosed and treated
Artificial flavors	Makes up for flavorless ingredients	Behavioral reactions and allergies	ADHD drugs, antihistamines
Artificial sweeteners	Stronger than sugar	90 reported symptoms, but commonly GI irritation, brain cancer, seizures, and migraines	Multiple types

Chemical	Purpose	Possible Health Damage or Symptom	Usual Treatment
High-fructose corn syrup	Cheaper than sugar, stimulates appetite	Extremely toxic to liver, increases inflammation, obesity, oxidative stress, and diabetes	You name it
Brominated vegetable oil (BVO)	Sports drink flavor emulsifier	Illegal in many countries. Competes with iodine, causing hypothyroidism, autoimmune diseases, and cancer.	Medicine treats symptoms
Blue 1, Blue 2, Yellow 5, Yellow 6	Coloring agents	Illegal in many countries. Made from coal tar. Used to kill certain bugs such as head lice.	No treatment
Olestra (Olean)	Fat-free products (potato chips)	Causes oily anal leakage. Interferes with fat-soluble vitamins. Banned in UK and Canada.	No treatment
Synthetic hormones	Increase milk production	Inhumane treatment of cows. Hormones enter the milk drinker, causing breast, colon, and prostate cancer.	
Arsenic	Improves efficiency in raising chickens and enhances meat color	Illegal in Europe. EPA classifies it as carcinogen.	Treat the disease it causes.

The list could go on for pages, but I just wanted to give a few examples to get you started. In other words, processing means removing nutrients, adding chemicals, increasing caloric content, and removing much of the fiber.

A great deal of information is available on this subject, including online, and it is worthy of study.

It's also important not to count on our government to protect us from these dangers. The more you take charge and learn which sources can be trusted to educate you about the food you eat, the better the chance you will have of enjoying a healthy, vital life. Some good sources are the Health Sciences Institute; the Conscious Life Project; the CBN News Health & Science website; and the Real Cures newsletter from Dr. Frank A. Shallenberger.

Prevention: Much Easier than Treatment

Prevention is so much easier than treating disease—but it is not for the lazy. Prevention means that you find out about what goes into the products you put into your body. New information is coming out so fast it's hard to follow, and our government is right in there with those wanting to profit from adding life-damaging substances to our food supply, allowing chemicals in our foods that are illegal in the foods of other countries. Most GMO products, for example, are illegal in many countries, yet our government not only allows them, but it appoints people from companies like Monsanto to the Environmental Protection Agency (EPA).

The beauty of the Paleo Diet is that it avoids all of the above poisons, as well as others not mentioned here. Just think, if you follow this diet, you miss out on all the misery that the processed-food consumer gets to enjoy! Yet many people, including the "experts" I quoted in previous chapters, say it's too hard to follow this diet. Let them enjoy their diet of processed foods, plus the prescribed medications they'll need to cover all the health dysfunction they'll experience as they age!

I only wish that this information had been available when I was young. Even after I was out of medical school, I suffered from believing what I had been taught. Nutrition at that time was for nutritionists. My philosophy was to enjoy things that tasted good. Oh, we knew that fattening things were bad and that butter should be replaced with margarine, and we knew to drink a lot of milk and eat a lot of grains (now the second-largest part of the USDA's Choose-MyPlate guidelines).

My reward was getting to have two hips replaced, plus heart surgery.

I now feel very strongly that—even though I have suffered considerable trauma, including broken bones—with my present lifestyle, those surgeries would not have been needed. At seventy-five, I feel better than I did at forty-five, and I'm enjoying a pain-free and energized life (no arthritis anywhere!) and writing this book.

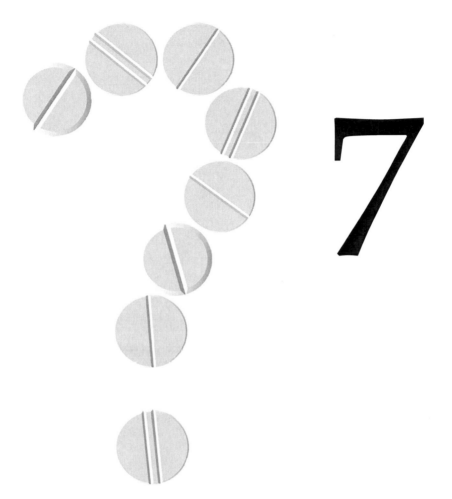

7

The Importance of
Supplementing Your Diet

The Importance of
Supplementing Your Diet

There's another area of diet that is traditionally swept under the rug or scoffed at by medical professionals: supplementation. Do you remember the World War II generals who wanted to continue to use horses? Well, in medicine they still exist. There continue to be self-proclaimed experts who criticize taking supplements. In fact, I was told in a nutrition course in dental school that I was very wrong to be taking 60 mg of vitamin C per day.

Today, while studying the use of supplements, I find doctors telling us that taking vitamins is not necessary if we're eating properly. What about farming properly? What about what is done to our food before we get it?

In 1938 the Public Health Service warned America that the continued use of the soil was depleting its minerals to the extent that vegetables might no longer be supplying what we needed. What has happened since? I have to buy glacier dust for my garden outside of California; someone won't allow it to be sold in the state because it contains asbestos.

Yes, serpentine, one of several rocks from which glacier dust is derived, is found throughout California, where I live—and it's where asbestos comes from. But I don't see people dying anywhere else that glacier dust exists. To the contrary, some of the healthiest people in the world live at high altitudes, where the water they drink and use for irrigation has glacier dust in it.

As pointed out in the chapter on diet and nutrition, many factors influence what actually enters our body. Sometimes a person just doesn't have what it takes to be able to get everything out of what he or she eats. Factors responsible for this are numerous, ranging from problems we're born with to self-inflicted damage, such as from the poisons we talked about in the previous chapter in processed foods, alcohol, and many more.

As I've pointed out, what you eat may be loaded with nutrition, but what gets into your blood may be quite different. Much of the time, it's necessary to add what is missing or add something that can make up for the damage our behavior has done to our digestive system.

There are many good doctors practicing holistic and alternative medicine. I highly recommend having a complete exam to determine how all of your body's systems are working. With proper guidance, many of the damaged organs and systems can be helped a lot. However, in this chapter, my goal is to propose normal supplementation, not the therapeutic dosages or approaches meant to heal damaged organs.

A complete organic diet, free from processed foods, is like giving medicine to your body. Even better is a good diet *plus* understanding what your body is deficient in.

Support for Supplementation

The following is a quote from an FDA statement on dietary supplements: "Unlike drugs, supplements *are not intended to treat, diagnose, prevent, or cure diseases.* This means supplements should not make claims, such as 'reduces arthritic pain' or 'treats heart disease.' Claims like these can only legitimately be made for drugs, not dietary supplements." I might add that only drug companies make drugs, and they heavily influence the FDA.

I challenge this statement. What about scurvy? Cured and prevented by vitamin C. What about rickets? Cured and prevented by vitamin D. What about pellagra? Cured and prevented by vitamin B3. Each year, usually during the summer, when kids are drinking sugar drinks like Kool-Aid, I see a lot of *angular chelitis*, which are chronic sores in the corner of their mouth. Sugar, a big source of empty calories, has caused the depletion of vitamin B6 from their bodies. Some doctors give them ointments, leaving the deficiency in place.

Many medical schools continue to give a very short, limited course on nutrition, and most of their students graduate lacking appreciation for its importance—to the point that I actually get criticized for recommending supplements.

A very famous cardiologist, Dr. Chauncey Crandall, feels that supplementation should be part of a heart-disease prevention program. On his list of supplements are niacin; folic acid; vitamins B1, B2, B6, B12, C, and D; coenzyme Q10; magnesium; hawthorn; and plant sterols.

This is very valid information. Each of us has

a unique body that may require a special pattern of supplementation, and it is best to be guided by an expert who has done a thorough analysis of your special needs. It's not a good idea to jump on a new idea or take something in which you are not deficient. There is a lot of hype on the Internet about various things being "special for you," but the vast majority of people who sell such supplements are motivated by greed, and such supplements will not help you at all; in fact, they could hurt.

When you do buy supplements, don't try to cut corners. Cheap vitamins can have a varnish on them to preserve them for testing. They exit the body in the same form as they entered it. Get direction from your health-care professional about the best sources to buy from, or have him or her supply supplements to you.

My help comes from a naturopathic endocrinologist who feels basic supplementation should include the following:

1. A probiotics, live strain (40–60 ppb) (once you're over forty)
2. Vitamin D3–4000 IU/day

(continued on next page)

3. A high-quality multimineral and
   multivitamin (minerals should be chelated)
4. High-quality fish oil (cheap oils can
   have toxic heavy metals)
5. An antioxidant blend

Don't fall for the normal instinct of thinking that if a little is good, a lot is better. Too much, especially of fat-soluble vitamins (A, D, E, and K), can be damaging. It wasn't until I corrected my lifestyle and eating habits, along with getting guidance, that I experienced incredible changes in my health and vitality.

I could never go back. No comfort food can replace feeling so good.

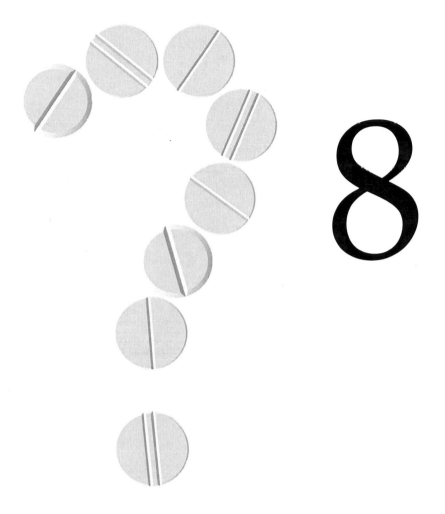

8

Legal Drug Abuse

Legal Drug Abuse

Now that we know how important it is to avoid substances that cause inflammation, let's look at one of the worst culprits: processed foods. They contain more than half of the inflammatory substances listed in the previous chapter—especially sugar and fat. And in order to turn your taste buds on, the food industry is not happy with just sugar and fat: they use high-fructose corn syrup and hydrogenated trans fats—which are even worse for your heart. In this case, the real motive is not just to preserve the food—it's greed (these products are cheaper).

In addition to understanding the relationship between diet and health, it's also critical to be aware of what is going on in the world of prescription drugs—and why we need to take responsibility for anything a doctor prescribes for us. In our symptom-focused medical model, prescribing a medication is the easy way for doctors to deal with their patients.

But as natural health expert Dr. Joseph Mercola stated in a 2011 article, "Death by medicine is a 21st-century epidemic, and America's 'war on drugs' is clearly directed at the wrong enemy!" He goes on to say that a 2009 analysis by the *Los Angeles Times* showed that for the first time ever in the United States, more people were killed by drugs than by motor vehicle accidents. And prescription drugs like OxyContin, Vicodin, and Xanax now cause more deaths than do heroine and cocaine combined. In fact, in an article published on October 25, 2013, the *New York Times* reported that 75 percent of drug-related deaths are caused by prescription drugs.

Always perform an Internet investigation of any prescription given to you by your doctor. You need to know why the drug is being given to you and, at the very least, what the drug's side effects are. I said "at the very least" because other factors can also change the effectiveness of a drug. Ask yourself the following questions about any drug you've been prescribed: Do I take it with food? Are there any foods or juices that interfere with its function? If I have several prescriptions, do they react with one another? Does the drug contribute to inflammation? (It would certainly help to have an inflammatory index for pharmaceuticals.) Also inquire if any another treatment could accomplish the desired goal, as in the case of using diet for arthritis and exercise for high blood pressure.

In some cases, such as with NSAIDS (nonsteroidal anti-inflammatory drugs), there are several classes of the drug. Each tends to have a limit on how long you can take it before it loses its effectiveness, at which point the class of NSAID needs to be changed.

In my TMJ clinic, I have had patients with over twenty prescriptions given by several doctors. My practice has a consultant, a PhD professor of pharmacology, who reviews my patients' drugs, most of the time finding that some interfere with each other and that some just aren't needed. Recent research has shown, for example, that NSAIDs can slow down healing. We have known for years that they can slow down orthodontic tooth movement.

When you consider that all drugs can have side effects, it is amazing some patients can function at all. It also makes you wonder what other drugs will be required down the road to treat the side effects of the current drugs in use.

One of the most common and profitable drugs prescribed is Lipitor. It's used to lower cholesterol, a much needed organic molecule called a sterol. Cholesterol plays a very important role in the body when the liver converts it to bile, which is necessary for the digestion of fats, without which we cannot live. The vitamins A, D, E, and K are all vitamins that require this.

Cholesterol is also required for the production of adrenal hormones, such as cortisol and aldosterone, and the sex hormones progesterone, estrogen, testosterone, and their derivatives. It also is an important factor in the formation of cell membranes.

The problem is that Lipitor is prescribed by specialists in cardiology. And your specialist might not understand what it's like for a man to lose his libido and become estrogenetic (female-hormone dominant, prone to prostate cancer).

Adding to the problem is one more piece of misinformation: some professionals have told me there are as many heart attacks with low cholesterol as there are with high. Too low cholesterol can also cause depression, cancer, stroke, erectile dysfunction, and prostate problems. But Lipitor itself can cause liver failure and death. *Always read about your prescription!*

I consider overuse of any drug to be drug abuse. If a doctor is not advising you about what nonpharmaceutical actions you can take to help your heart, for example, you are not being given all the information you really need. Now that inflammation has been found to be an important factor in heart disease, does he or she have you on antioxidants and a diet that fights inflammation? Are you continuing to eat foods made with trans fats? Has he or she warned you that you must avoid inflammatory foods and habits? Does he or she even know about these very important factors? I have yet to find a cardiac patient who has been given enough information on these matters.

Another specialty in medicine, rheumatology, deals with arthritis, but it tends to ignore why the patient is ill and treat only symptoms. Steroids are given for the inflammation, NSAIDs and narcotics for the pain, and gold injections to slow down the progress of the disease.

At lunch today, a good friend was complaining about her arthritic pain, and because I practice in a related field, she asked if I would prescribe her meds. I had to tell her I rarely use meds. If my patients follow my instructions, they don't need them except in the case of a severe crisis.

She told me her doctor said arthritis is not curable and not to pay attention to all that nonsense about diet and supplements. I recommended changing doctors to one with a more holistic view of health and the human body.

Dr. Collin Dong was one such doctor. He published the book *New Hope for the Arthritic* in 1976. An American-trained and American-licensed MD, his treatment for arthritis consisted primarily of changes to diet and lifestyle. This treatment was responsible for arresting thousands of very serious cases of all types of arthritis. Yes, he did prescribe medications, but his goal was for patients to take them at a minimum and hopefully end use of all drugs.

I first became aware of Dr. Dong when a therapist who worked in my office related her story to me. She had been crippled with rheumatoid arthritis and had gone to him out of desperation.

As long as she was strict and held to his prescribed plan, she was able to enjoy life and follow her passion as a ski instructor on the weekends.

Dr. Dong's book should be required reading for all doctors and therapists who treat arthritics. And since this book was written, even more foods to avoid for arthritis have been discovered. Could it be that there is an awful lot of money to be made in selling arthritis drugs? Does the influence the drug industry has over universities lead to an emphasis on the use of drugs instead of alternatives?

There will always be those patients who want a quick fix, with no responsibility other than taking pills. I can't blame the doctors who give such patients pills, but when those doctors say nutritional methods don't work, they're violating their oath to first do no harm. Their overmedicated patients will possibly suffer many diseases as a result of the side effects of these drugs. In addition, many foods have been proven to increase arthritic symptoms, causing decreased effects of the drugs and requiring higher doses or additional medications.

Today, in my clinic, I had a patient tell me she couldn't follow Dr. Dong's recommendations because she didn't like vegetables, didn't like having regular meals, and, as far as I could see, didn't like most things that are required to be healthy.

I feel very fortunate that my treatment worked for her TMJ, but she has arthritis pain throughout her body and would rather take narcotics than take any helpful steps that might require her to avoid the processed garbage she lives on.

Thank God most of my patients are not like this, or I might have been tempted to treat just the symptoms, and with so little reward, I would probably be retired and playing golf by now. I would definitely have a lot more money if I had supported such laziness—but it's not the path I chose.

Drugs Treating Symptoms

In chapter 2, we talked about the problem of treating symptoms only—never getting to the root cause of disease. Let's look now at some examples of this in various fields of medicine, particularly the role that drugs typically play in treatments for these various problems.

OTORHINOLARYNGOLOGY (Ear, Nose, Throat—ENT). It's common to place tubes in the ears of a child suffering from chronic ear infections, usually following an attempt to control such infections with decongestants and antibiotics. However, like so many other health problems we've already discussed, a common cause of this disease is dairy food allergies. A large percentage of children are allergic to dairy foods. In my orthodontic practice, when parents want to help their children, removing dairy from their diet can solve the problem. Dairy can also be the cause of problems with large tonsils and adenoids.

Not treating the cause can result in a congested airway, a major factor altering the growth and development of the face and dental structures. Recent research has demonstrated that nasal breathing is very important to one's health, even influencing cardiac variability, one of the characteristics of good heart health.

DERMATOLOGY. There are many examples of treating symptoms in this area, but I will limit this discussion to acne. Many, many drugs and medicines are used to hide the symptoms—pimples—while it would be so much better to get at the cause. Again, one of the most common causes is dairy. For some reason, in our country, condemning milk is like condemning God! Where is my child going to get calcium? Well, again I ask, where does the cow get it? From vegetables!

Throughout my forty-nine years of practicing orthodontics, I've seen a lot of teenagers with acne. Although I've taken a lot of flak from the many members of the "church of milk" as well as from uninformed doctors, I have had consistent success helping my patients out of this difficult stage. In fact, I can't count the number of teens I've helped through this ugly stage of life.

The most dangerous drug I've seen used for acne is Accutane. It is so bad, it can cause birth defects if a girl becomes pregnant while using it. Recent research has demonstrated that it negatively affects the production of telomerase, the major enzyme mentioned previously that affects gene reproduction, prevents cancer, and slows aging. Who knows what we will find when the Accutane generation ages? When you look at all the other side effects, if I didn't know what motivates the FDA, I would wonder why they have allowed this drug—and still do.

And have you heard the ads for the drugs to treat psoriasis? They describe unbelievable side effects in using these drugs to hide symptoms often caused by gluten sensitivity.

UROLOGY AND ERECTILE DYSFUNCTION (ED). Thank the drug gods for Cialis, Viagra, and Levitra. Forget the cause of ED. It could be another medicine he is taking, heart disease, hormone imbalance, alcoholism, or any number of problems, but he will be happy tonight and smiling tomorrow, and the doctor and insurance companies will be much healthier financially.

The urologist is the specialist who treats such problems as ED and prostate cancer. If urologists and cardiologists could get together, it might be possible to handle the heart without destroying the man. The drug companies wouldn't like this, though, for they love one drug to cause the need for another.

ONCOLOGY. Chemotherapy and radiation are the most commonly used treatments for cancer. Yet no one should be proud of the results, including the damage, the pain, and the misery of the treatments. I've lost my mother, father, and sister, as well as many friends, to cancer. Thank God for hospice.

In 1925, Dr. Otto Warburg first wrote of his findings; he was awarded the Nobel Prize in 1931. In a previous chapter, I noted that he discovered two major causes of cancer: lack of blood oxygen and low blood alkalinity. Evidence has suggested that if a person can achieve good oxygen and higher blood alkalinity levels, his or her cancer risk is much less. Societies that have a diet and lifestyle providing this have little or no cancer.

One such treatment is the simple, cheap chemical cesium chloride, which has been used to alkalize the blood, arresting cancer and effecting a cure. But doctors who have attempted to apply these ideas to the treatment of cancer have been stopped by our FDA and, in some cases, incarcerated.

Blood oxygenation, sometimes using ozone, has also been very successful. But most of the time, you must leave the country to get these treatments. READ! There is much information on the Internet and in the literature—I've come across numerous journals and books while researching—regarding the many sources of alternative medicine that are curing cancer without chemo and radiation.

I hope you aren't seeing an oncologist, but in many cases, such a doctor would say the above is nonsense—you must accept our poor results and enjoy the misery that goes along with our conventional treatments.

Yesterday I was at a Halloween party for dental offices. A wonderful lady dentist was sitting beside me and related that she had had to take a break from practice due to the side effects of chemotherapy. Noticing she was eating several Halloween treats, I asked if she were aware that cancer loves sugar. Of course the answer was no. Apparently, her doctor didn't have the slightest knowledge of the cause of the disease he was specialized to treat. Such negligence meant he was not giving his patient the best chance to survive.

• • •

What I have gone over in this chapter just touches the surface of what a medical society controlled by the pharmaceutical industry—and "evidence-based" and "standard-of-care" thinking—has become. If you look at the reality of "evidence-based" logic, the evidence is overwhelming that many of their methods aren't working.

As I've mentioned, a great percentage of patients in our society want the quick and easy way of symptom relief and never want to have to be a part of the solution. We need typical doctors for them—and there are too many ready to help.

But my reason for writing this book is to reach out to those of you who want the best care possible and are willing to participate proactively in your treatment—so you can get it!

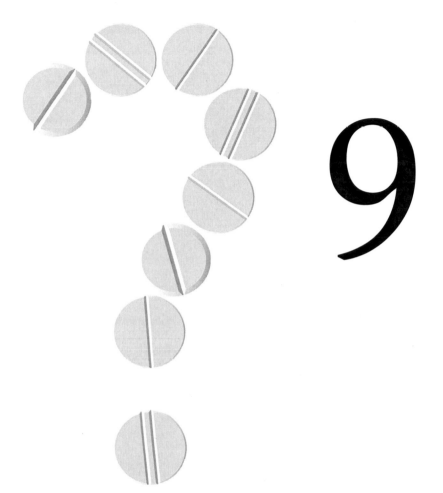

9

Acupuncture:
The Rise of Complementary
and Alternative Medicine

Acupuncture: The Rise of Complementary and Alternative Medicine

In 1998, Congress established the National Center for Complementary and Alternative Medicine (NCCAM). It was an important step in a system that is slow to embrace "outside-the-box" thinking, and it was encouraging to see the rise of the CAM movement. According to an article on WebMD, by 1990, a third of Americans had used some form of CAM, which includes therapies and practices such as yoga, meditation, massage, and herbal medicine. That number had doubled by 2002, and it continues to rise.

One of the most astonishing of these alternative therapies that I have witnessed and personally experienced is the ancient practice of acupuncture in place of our conventional use of anesthesia for surgery. Following is an interview with Dr. Paul Dudley White (who has been called the Father of American Cardiology), taken from the *Boston Herald-Journal,* October 31, 1971. Dr. White had just returned from mainland China, where he was impressed with what he had observed regarding this practice.

Q: *Did you witness surgery with acupuncture?*

A: Yes. We did see surgery in the totally new thing of using acupuncture as the only anesthetic. I wouldn't have believed it possible. We saw to our satisfaction that the Chinese surgeons weren't faking it—I am quite sure the patients had no preparatory drugs ahead of acupuncture, except for the rare tranquilizer. They were awake and quite alert during the operations.

Several hospitals we visited displayed surgery with acupuncture—on purpose, I think, to elicit our interest in helping to determine how it works. For the Chinese say they don't know either.

Q: *What type of operations did you witness?*

A: We saw three patients have vigorous tooth extractions with only an acupuncture needle stuck into a jaw, or firm pressure over such a point. One 10-year-old boy immediately afterward shook hands with us and ran off.

We watched a woman whose skull had been opened for removal of a brain tumor, and I talked with her, through an interpreter, of course, with her skull lying open. It was incredible. We saw a man having an upper lobe of his lung removed and a woman operated upon for removal of an ovarian cyst.

Q: *What is the technique, or techniques, of acupuncture?*

A: The needles don't need to be near the area being operated on. Putting them between the tendons of the right wrist seemed to be a favorite location that we witnessed. Sometimes the acupuncturist twisted the needles during surgery. Maybe this is a bit painful and distracts the patient. Sometimes they sent a small electrical charge through the needle.

Q: Do you have ideas about how acupuncture may be successful in this way of being an anesthetic?

A: No, not really. Grey Diamond, a distinguished professor of medicine at the University of Missouri-Kansas City, says he plans to start research into the matter. . . . One man, after the removal of a thyroid adenoma (cancer), climbed off the operating table, shook hands with us, and walked away. For one thing, the patients seemed to have few or no post-operative complications common after general anesthesia. They could often eat a light meal directly after the operation.

Please keep in mind that this interview was done over forty-two years ago, but that acupuncture is yet to be considered a "standard of care."

I saw a video on this subject done by Dr. White and associates in the early 1970s. I was so impressed that I attended a course in acupuncture in 1973 at UCLA—and personally had acupuncture performed on me to relieve severe pain several years ago when I was in an accident. Both shoulders were broken in that accident, along with my upper jaw and front teeth.

The thing about me is that, once intense pain has subsided, I cannot stand narcotics. So in this case, in addition to many other needles, an acupuncture needle was placed on the bridge of each foot, instantly relieving the pain in the broken shoulders, with no side effects.

I have had a great deal of success referring my pain patients out for such treatment.

This is just one more reason for my desire to write this book. Why is our medical establishment so reluctant to acknowledge that there is often a better way? General anesthesia used to prepare a prisoner for the death penalty has been judged as cruel and unusual. So why do we use it on even minor surgeries? A friend of mine lost his wife due to the anesthesia used for a simple plastic-surgery procedure.

It can take days to eliminate the poisons used to induce anesthesia, and there is the chance that the side effects can be prolonged or even permanent. Doesn't it sound better to get off the operating table and walk to your hospital bed than to be wheeled back on a gurney to a recovery room to wait for the poison to dissipate?

Is there a shred of compassion and concern for the misery and potentially life-threatening results that this field of medicine provides? As mentioned in chapter 1 on left- and right-brained thinking, those doctors lacking in balance between the two tend to be the self-proclaimed leaders and politicians in medicine. Unfortunately, they will be the ones to decide what medicine does.

Failure to recognize and accept alternative therapies such as acupuncture seems to be a function of another left-brain characteristic: the reluctance to allow new ideas—especially not scientifically proven, "evidence-based" ideas—to be considered in one's practice. Acupuncture has been around for over six thousand years. That is a great deal more evidence than "modern" medicine can offer. There is a clever statement commonly heard in medical schools: "Those who can do, do, and those who can't do, teach." Thank God this is not true of all professors!

It is more than apparent that the greed of the pharmaceutical industry and some of those in the medical industry far outweighs any desire to do what is best for the patient. Why have there not been billions of dollars spent on research to find out why acupuncture works? Can you imagine the new discoveries that would occur in researching such a unique field of medicine, which we know almost nothing about and yet which works?

By studying what causes something to work so well when science cannot explain why, entirely new fields of medicine would form, and new knowledge of what makes our bodies work could help answer many present mysteries. Our present medical establishment should be ashamed of such neglect. Acupuncture is a therapy that works, yet when medical leaders can't figure out why, their attitude is to throw it out. Is that intelligence or just an "evidence-based" junkie's way of thinking?

Knowing what makes acupuncture work just might force the FDA to approve its use. But it is quite evident that this is not their desire. Look at all the anesthesiologists who would be out of work and the losses that would be incurred by the pharmaceutical industry and medical equipment industries if acupuncture were approved. Even hospital bills would be lower. Everyone would lose—except the patient!

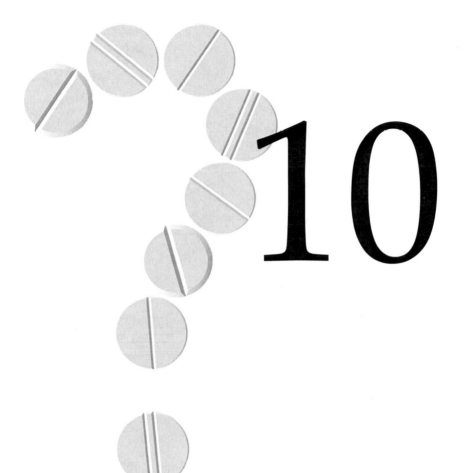

*Epidemiology: A Proposal
to Save Billions and
End Suffering*

Epidemiology: A Proposal to Save Billions and End Suffering

E pidemiology is the study of disease distribution in populations, a powerful tool for understanding and addressing the underlying causes of disease. Yet this science has gone neglected and underdeveloped for decades. Let's take a closer look at what it involves and how it might be used to the great benefit of all our citizens.

Epidemiology focuses on groups, rather than individuals, and often includes a historical perspective. *Descriptive epidemiology* surveys a population to see what segments (e.g., age, sex, ethnic group, occupation) are affected by a disorder, follows changes or variations in the disorder's incidence or mortality rate over time and in different locations, and helps identify syndromes or suggest associations with risk factors.

Analytic epidemiology conducts studies to

test the conclusions of descriptive surveys or laboratory observations. Epidemiologic data on diseases is used to find those at high risk, identify causes, take preventive measures, and plan new health services.

So why is epidemiology overlooked? Could it be that someone would lose great sums of money if the causes of some diseases were discovered and symptom-treating medications were no longer necessary?

It seems unbelievable that a government that has spent billions building monstrous facilities to gather personal information on you and me—to possibly save a few hundred lives that might be lost through terrorism—cannot apply an effort to save millions of us from debilitating and fatal diseases.

A National Database for National Health

I propose that we standardize medical histories for all doctor and hospital patients and enter them into a national database. Each history could be transmitted to a central national database without the name of the patient on it, but coded so that follow-up medical histories and symptoms could be added.

Even better would be a scenario in which millions volunteered to be in the data bank, name and all. If the histories were complete—including dietary habits, exercise habits, and environmental factors, as well as the regular questions—science could find many common factors leading to a disease, possibly ending its occurrence.

For example, the cause of diseases such as Lou Gehrig's disease (ALS) remains a mystery, although the incidence is higher in Gulf War veterans. To contact every person with the disease and search for something in common, such as exposure to chemicals used on grass or in the jungles, would cost so little.

Another example might be the incidence of ear infections in babies. Was the child nursed? Did the mother drink cow's milk while nursing? What foods was the baby fed? As I've noted, in my practice, the elimination of dairy products reduces a great percentage of recurrent ear infections and often considerably reduces the size of the tonsils and adenoids.

I am the father of four children. Two were allergic to dairy. The two who drank milk had to have tonsillectomies. The lucky ones who were allergic did not develop large tonsils.

With the medical histories available from millions of patients suffering from the same disease—what was done, what worked, and what the side effects were—the information would be right there for all to know, and new, more successful treatments could be developed. These facts are going unused and could dramatically reduce pain and suffering, disease, and death.

The results of gathering this vital information could also be used to measure the incidence of the side effects of the use of a medication. If a great percentage of patients taking an arthritis drug go to another practitioner for gastric reflux disease, and this is documented and reported to the medical profession and available to the public, then changes in the use of the drug might be made. But these reports would have to be made public.

This is such a logical approach. Why should you have to search the Internet and literature to uncover the obvious, which could be easily revealed by overwhelming statistics?

The beauty of epidemiology, properly done, is that the resulting reports are facts. This medication is taken for this symptom, and these are the results of what others have experienced. What happened to those who did nothing and got well also? If a pregnant woman takes this drug or uses this substance, the chances of birth defects are X%, and these defects are (fill in the blank). Now we rely on the drug companies to supply this information. Is it possible there's a conflict of interest here?

As these forms of reporting are perfected, even lifestyles and dietary habits can be analyzed to report to us how these and other factors create misery in our old age. It will take years to develop this field, but even the simplest medical history of millions can tell us enough to be significant right now. In addition, I have enough faith in Americans to propose that many would voluntarily fill out forms to help create data banks that could be of extreme importance.

I don't think there would be great financial losses to the food industries or pharmaceutical industries if such information were to become available to us. The vast majority of the public won't make the effort to change and become proactive in their health. Such information would simply make it possible for those of us who want optimal health to have the facts we'd need. However, doctors would be forced to revise their stands when the facts overwhelmingly disagreed with their beliefs, such as in the case of diet and arthritis.

As I mentioned earlier, to help all better understand health topics and prevent injury to our bodies, I propose the teaching of physiology from K through 12. It is hard to understand why this has never been done. Here we are—born with a body we have to take care of and live in for a lifetime—and we don't even have an owner's manual!

Even when we do know about the potentially harmful effects of doing certain things to our bodies, we often think we're immune. I see so many teenagers smoking, knowing full well the damage it does. None of my children smoke, but they grew up making me a promise that, if they ever did, they would allow me to take them to my medical school and open up a cadaver's chest to show them the tar deposits. Then I would also take them to see patients recovering from surgery for lung cancer.

I mentioned earlier that I used to teach some local fourth grade classes the dangers of smoking and chewing. I had some nasty, graphic slides and testimonies from baseball players, with photos of the mouth cancer they suffered. This was but one hour on one day of the school year, but the students went home and raised hell with their smoking parents and chewing siblings.

Can you imagine the power these kids would have to control their health if they were given one hour every day to learn about that precious gift we've been given? Of course, there would be many who would continue to destroy themselves, but it would no longer be due to society's neglect.

One problem with this idea is that there aren't big profits to be made in educating ourselves to maintain good health, nor a big enough amount of money to convince politicians and bureaucrats to support a large-scale change in the way we approach health. Without fulfilling the greed requirements of our society, it is really difficult to get such a project off the ground.

And once the information is there for those who care, there will always be those who don't care. Today I was talking to someone who has a friend with multiple sclerosis (MS). Though she's crippled and forced to use a walker, no one has mentioned to her the importance of avoiding certain foods. Part of her country's tradition is a special dough fried in vegetable oil and served for breakfast. The rest of her diet is horrible, but, although the information is there, it would take effort for her doctor to suggest changes, and there wouldn't be any profit in doing so.

Yes, epidemiology would be invaluable to health care, potentially saving billions in treatment costs and preventing endless pain and suffering. But getting someone to learn and apply this information is another story. That is why I feel so strongly that you must play a big part in demanding the best.

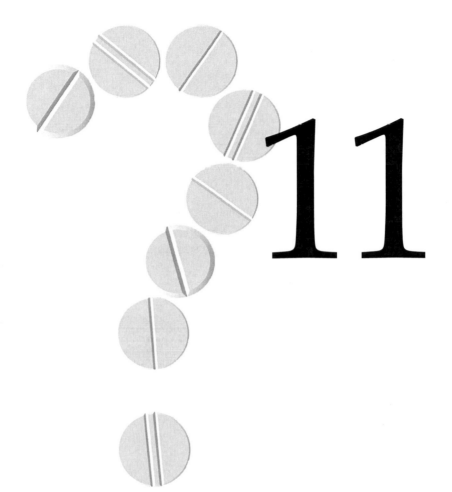

11

Why Do We Have to Fight the Government?

Why Do We Have to
Fight the Government?

Greed is one of the single most motivating factors for any action in our society, not only in our political community, but among the public as well. Greed takes many forms, from the love of money, to the lust for power, to the desire to get something for nothing quickly. It has been a very, very long time since our government was "of the people, by the people, for the people." Now it seems to be more "of the demagogues, by the demagogues, for the demagogues."

The definition of demagogy is "the art and practice of gaining power and popularity by arousing the emotions, passions, and prejudices of the people." Elected politicians don't seem to want to represent the needs and interests of the electorate anymore—they want to own the electorate for their gain.

To make matters worse, demagogy dominates the media, which works hard to cover for themselves and their political cohorts.

Among the various agencies of the government, there seems almost to be a competition to see which agency can outdo the others in violating our rights and neglecting our needs. Right now the competition is strong between the Food and Drug Administration (FDA), the Internal Revenue Service (IRS), and the Environmental Protection Agency (EPA). All are acting so far outside the law that their practices, if done in a nongovernment business, would put their executives in jail. Insider trading is one of the many areas of the law in which you and I would face criminal charges with severe sentences, while members of our Congress get rich doing it.

However, in the interest of keeping this book nonpolitical, I will concentrate on the actions of just one of these agencies: the tremendous effort and expense the FDA has applied to preventing successful treatment of cancer, as in the case of Dr. Stanislaw Burzynski.

Question: How did our government ever allow lobbyists into the FDA? That is similar to allowing lobbyists for the jury in a court case. Does the FDA really need input from a drug company to become knowledgeable enough to make a decision?

Here is an example of their misbehavior. Dr. Burzynski, an MD and PhD biochemist, runs a clinic in Texas where he has developed a method of treating cancer based on antineoplastons. Cancer cells have different genes from those of normal cells. Dr. Burzynski discovered that antineoplastons are able to target these genes specifically, rather than grossly targeting all cells—thus possibly killing the cancer before chemotherapy kills the patient.

This is particularly true of brain cancer, where chemo and radiation do so much damage to the brain that the patient usually dies, or at least becomes blind and deaf. By targeting the cells with different genes, only the cancer cells are destroyed, and the patient has a much better chance of survival.

When and if this treatment is finally approved, it will mark a first in history. No scientist has ever developed an exclusive patent on a paradigm-shifting medical breakthrough without being part of a pharmaceutical industry.

But so far, the FDA has rewarded Dr. Burzynski with a total of five grand-jury indictments, with potential penalties upon conviction totaling 290 years in jail and $18.5 million in fines. Thank God the courts in his cases weren't owned by the big pharmaceutical industry. In all cases, he was found not guilty. But the harassment went on for more than fourteen years.

Presently, the FDA continues to harass Dr. Burzynski by approving his treatment in the first two of three stages but making it impossible to pass stage III. His methods are so different from current practices that they cannot comply with FDA standards. So just who are these "standards" protecting?

I highly recommend going to the website www.burzynskimovie.com (the movie is also on YouTube). If you are going to be proactive in achieving optimal health, this is a must-see film.

The next example of this type of corruption is the case of the Milan mutation. A rare protein was discovered in the small town of Limone sul Garda in Italy. The following article was released in the U.S. *Department of Energy Science News* in 2002:

*May 28, 2002—Lawrence Berkeley National-
al Laboratory researchers have discovered the
mechanism by which an extremely rare protein
mutation shields people from cardiovascular disease. The mutation enables the protein to curb
oxidation, a harmful process in which molecules
with unpaired electrons, also called free radicals,
scavenge electrons from healthy tissue. It's believed to play a role in such diverse diseases as
Alzheimer's, osteoporosis, and a form of heart
disease known as atherosclerosis.*

*In atherosclerosis, free radicals grab electrons
from lipids that line artery walls, sparking an
inflammatory response that paves the way for
cholesterol deposition. The mutated protein,
however, boasts an antioxidant in the form of a
sulfur-based residue that mops up unpaired electrons and prevents them from triggering arterial
inflammation, according to John K. Bielicki of
Berkeley Lab's Life Sciences Division.*

*This time a drug company intervened, buy-
ing up the rights to apoA-I, and changed the
name to MDCO-216. Research had been going
well and there was so much excitement that it
was covered by 60 Minutes and reported in the
Journal of the American Medical Association in*

November of 2003. Pfizer bought up the rights to apoA-I by buying Esperion Therapeutics and shut down research, while they made a fortune on Lipitor.

As we discussed in an earlier chapter, Lipitor is among the biggest money-making drugs ever to hit the market. It is a statin drug that lowers cholesterol, but it really hasn't been proven beyond doubt to prevent heart disease. It does, however, have side effects that cannot only take away the joy in life, for men in particular, but can also be fatal. Cholesterol is an important part of our cell membranes. Hormones such as testosterone, progesterone, and estrogen are cholesterols, as are all steroids. Altering these hormone levels can lead to numerous negative side effects.

Back when I trusted medicine, I was given Lipitor. It took years to overcome some of the side effects.

Recently there was an article entitled "Pros and Cons of Statins for Your Heart" in a report called *Everyday Health*. It was a typical Western medical approach: nowhere was there any mention of alternative treatments. Of course, the

"Milano mutation" has somehow disappeared into oblivion in the USA. Some work is still being done in Europe, but it seems that so many of these well-intentioned researchers are so locked into the "standard of care" that, not only can they not get outside the box, but the box has been bolted and chained.

Maybe many of the researchers look at what Burzynski went through and feel the fear of the FDA "god." To make matters worse, in each state there are demagogues who are either on the take or just plain prejudiced and who attempt to penalize doctors and practitioners who step outside the box. A pioneer of ozone therapy, for example, was forced to leave California and practice in Nevada. Now ozone therapy is accepted treatment for certain maladies, and a society of medical ozone therapists has been formed.

In California the "standard of care" for loss of cartilage in the knee used to be knee replacement, which can have many complications and is quite painful. But if you crossed the border into Nevada, you could get Prolozone therapy, replacing the cartilage noninvasively with your own cartilage.

The courts use the "standard of care" in your area to make decisions in malpractice judgments, so that a judge and jury with absolutely no knowledge can decide the outcome of such a lawsuit. Our system will not even allow a knowledgeable person such as a doctor or scientist to be on the jury. I have had the displeasure of being an expert witness trying to explain medical conditions to a judge who did not even understand the language.

The last example of federal interference goes back more than eighty-five years to 1925, when Dr. Otto Warburg introduced his findings that alkaline blood and oxygen kill cancer. As I mentioned earlier, in 1931 he was given the Nobel Prize for these discoveries. But for decades, and even now, treatment using these findings is not the standard of care, and practitioners have even been incarcerated for attempting to use these treatments.

A close friend of mine recently found it necessary to go to Mexico to a clinic of American doctors to be treated. He is alive and active as a result of these "illegal treatments." These treatments do not use hideously expensive drugs and do not have the horrible side effects either, but they don't line the pockets of those running the show, which may be why they're not allowed in the United States.

The following is a short report from the sister of a woman who used Dr. Warburg's methods, as reported in an article entitled "Dr. Otto Warburg and How to Kill Cancer Cells" on the website NeuroTalk.com:

My sister last year was given 2 years to live if she took chemo and radiation, and she did not because our mother, grandmother and grandfather, and almost the entire mother's side of the family had passed away with cancer. She tried alternative therapy and was recently dismissed as a cancer patient from the oncologist. Reason: they could not find any trace of cancer in her body. Please read! My sister is alive because she read with an open mind.

In order to slightly curb the demagogy that exists in our culture, we should demand a constitutional amendment that requires all members of federal and state governments to live by the same laws we do. Too many bureaucrats have too much power over our personal lives, and we have too little recourse. When you add political correctness to the pot, further obstructions get in the way of truth.

Neither politics nor greed—nor anything interfering with truth and fact—should have a place in medicine and health care. The opposite has been the rule for too long, and you and I have to do something to reverse the course. Yet we must all find a way to help; otherwise, these practices will continue or even grow.

I recently heard a clever phrase: "If you don't give them your two cents' worth, how can you expect change?" This book is part of my contribution.

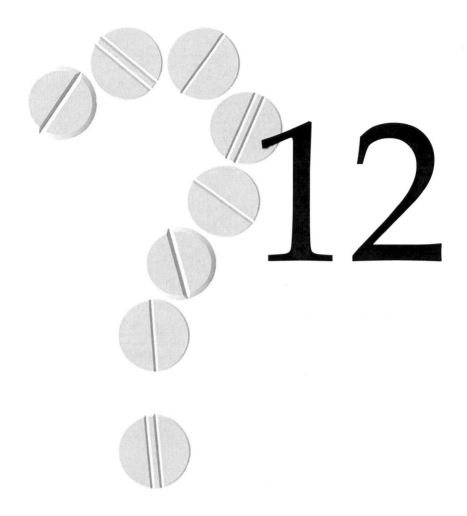

12

What Can YOU Do to Help?

What Can YOU Do to Help?

As I've mentioned several times, many doctors are so used to patients who want a "quick fix"—probably most—that as soon as those doctors hear the symptom you've come in with, they're thinking of a drug to hide that symptom. Or because it is the standard of care, those doctors might order a lab test, x-ray, or MRI.

If you're one of the "quick fix" devotees, you'll be lucky, because your doctor will save you time and write a prescription then and there. Off you'll go, and shortly after that, the pain or symptom will be gone.

There are those in our society who hate holistic medicine. When they go to see a doctor for a symptom, they don't want to look any further—they just want the symptom treated. This happened to me last week. A patient complained of jaw pain, inability to open her mouth more than one inch, and migraine headaches. She didn't like all the questions she had to answer.

When I touched acupuncture point C1, she felt pain. But she was furious when I mentioned the possibility of a colon irritation and the possible need to refer her for colon therapy. It was also painful, though necessary, when I took an impression for an orthotic splint.

I've been doing this for thirty-five years with a very high success rate. But this patient went straight to her referral source and filed a formal complaint—and will never come back. Fortunately, incidents like this are few and far between, and they don't get me down because I have the gratitude of thousands of patients who have been cured.

How You Can Be Proactive with Your Health

For those of you who want to be proactive in your treatment and seek out a cure for the underlying cause of your disease, there are many things you can do to help yourselves:

- Go on the Internet and research what could possibly be going on. You might just find that your doctor is impressed with your knowledge and will at least either explain to you why you are misinformed or congratulate you on your understanding of the problem. This is the sign of a good doctor.

- Arrive early at your doctor's office so that you have time to fill out the medical history and chief complaint forms in detail. Encourage the doctor to review your history by bringing up some of the things that are important to you. Make sure the reason for your visit is clearly explained, including the circumstances associated with the first signs of your complaint.

- In my practice, this part is quite important. Is it worse at night, when you wake, or after exercise or stress? The smallest detail can change everything in the diagnosis. A migraine headache can be due to an irritated bowel; in fact, one study at a pain clinic found that over 80 percent of migraine diagnoses were not really migraines.

- Be honest and open. Hiding something can only hurt and interfere with your treatment. You are not the only one who has had something bad happen to you or who has done something he or she would rather not talk about. It has recently been discovered that things that happened in our childhoods—a concussion, severe illness, or emotional or physical trauma—can all create problems that return later to haunt us. One example is that the stress caused by child abuse can severely damage one's telomeres, resulting in accelerated aging and predisposition to cancer and other diseases. Medicine is on the verge of being able to reverse this damage, thanks to the discovery of telomerase and how to stimulate its production.

- Attempt to find out if the doctor is capable of thinking outside the box. How does he or she feel about holistic or alternative medicine? Can nutrition be a factor? What about food combining? What about processed and genetically altered foods? Do supplements work? What about herbs?

- What does he or she think about acupuncture? Don't ask all these questions, but if he says anything is worthless when you are aware of the value, it's time to be on guard. I know of a rheumatologist who told a friend of mine who suffers from rheumatoid arthritis that nutrition was not a factor in that disease. I could never trust in his ability to treat me.

- When you are given a prescription, ask about the side effects of that drug. If your doctor is unaware of them, go home and look them up on the Internet. I want my doctor to be an expert on the medicine he wants me to take. For many doctors, the only knowledge of the medication comes from the detail man who introduced it to the practice, and he definitely won't try to warn the doctor against prescribing it.

- Follow the doctor's orders all the way. If the sleep medicine doctor finds that you have obstructive sleep apnea (OSA) and tells you to lose weight, try to lose weight. If the cardiologist wants you to exercise, do it. If you are lucky enough to have a doctor who is interested in your nutrition and eating habits, become knowledgeable in that area and correct those habits.

• Begin your own study of what makes your body what it is. I have to warn you that there are a lot of writers out there who write more opinion than fact. But thanks to the Internet, you can learn enough to really make your life incredibly vital and healthy. Yes, at times, it will be quite a challenge to say no to things that aren't good for you. But as I mentioned earlier, part of my diet includes an occasional splurge, like a prime rib dinner with a great dessert. The reward is worth it when you're seventy-five, look more like fifty-five, are able to do things some can't do at forty-five, and emotionally feel thirty-five!

In most circumstances, when a patient is given a program to follow, he or she tells me it's too hard. I remind him or her that everything truly valuable and rewarding in life is difficult to achieve. But most of the people who won't do things because the effort is too much then go through life regretting and complaining. The fact that what I want my patients to do seems hard should be a signal to be thankful for the opportunity to achieve the ultimate reward.

If you persist in following a proper diet, soon your body will start telling you when you're being poisoned. I get a backache about half an hour after eating gluten. If you persist in a good exercise regime, when you first start, it's hard and tiring. But keep it up, and soon it will not only be easy but enjoyable and rewarding.

Read as much as you can on health subjects, especially about how to control stress and your emotions to create happiness within you. Try to keep up on progress in medicine, new discoveries, and ideas to improve the way you live. If you hear about a new supplement, research it. Just like the pharmaceutical industry, the producers of supplements not only want to sell you as much as possible, but they'll sometimes sneak you onto an auto-order program.

Certain supplements are quite harmful taken in larger doses. All of the fat-soluble vitamins (A, D, E, and K) are poison in large doses. Excessive antioxidants are thought to have possible harmful effects too. If someone suggests something to you that isn't found in nature, check it out first. I find it quite enjoyable studying health topics on the Internet, in published newsletters, and in books. As you become more knowledgeable, you'll be able to spot the ample amounts of misinformation to be found on the Internet and in the literature.

Too many pseudo-scientists have never been exposed to the discipline of scientific writing and are merely expressing an opinion. These writers tend to believe that, if it is published, it's true. Be skeptical of an article about a big, new breakthrough claiming to be a miracle product and a panacea for all health problems.

Having a health-care specialist, especially a holistic one you can go to with questions about health products, helps a lot. Years ago my dermatologist gave me a steroid cream for what was probably psoriasis. I dropped by my naturopath's office and asked about this treatment. Her answer was to stop eating gluten.

It changed my life.

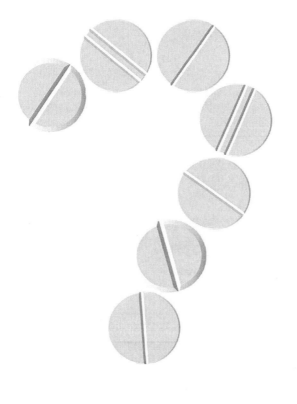

CONCLUSION

CONCLUSION

Imagine yourself feeling the best you have ever felt, appearing younger than you did five years ago, with no fear of colds and flu. Once you achieve this goal, would you ever want to go back? Once you begin to give yourself what it takes to keep a fulfilling life going, it becomes much easier to do what some feel is impossible: clean up your lifestyle nutritionally and emotionally—long after others have committed to slowing down and giving up.

How I Do It

Many people ask what my normal day looks like. I'm one of the lucky people who doesn't have to commute; I live ten minutes from my office. My day starts at 6:30 a.m. with a 15- to 20-minute Tobata-style workout, where you give it your all for 20 seconds, then rest for 10 seconds.

I'm fortunate that my workout is guided by my youngest daughter, a physical fitness trainer.

This type of exercise is similar to the Tibetan Five Rites exercises; it imitates a more normal human activity than do many other methods. Extended cardio exercise has actually been proven to harm the heart.

For breakfast, I always eat organic, gluten-free and dairy-free meals. I like either cage-free eggs; freshly made vegetable juice with some of the pulp; hot oatmeal with lightly stewed berries; or tropical fruit, such as mangoes and papayas. I love freshly ground organic coffee. Morning supplements are a probiotic, resveratrol, a vitamin-mineral complex, and vitamin D3.

My favorite lunch is a large salad, which includes several greens, steamed vegetables, nuts, and berries, with an olive oil dressing topped with grilled chicken or ahi. My midday supplements are CoQ10 and green tea.

Dinner I keep simple: one or two vegetables and a small piece of white meat. Being mostly French, I also include a very nice glass or two of wine with dinner. I always prepare my own breakfast and dinner, but once a week, I go out for sushi. My evening supplement is an omega-3 (when I don't have fish) and, before bed, chelated magnesium and melatonin.

Notice there was no mention of snacks or desserts. They are saved for special occasions. I do splurge once or twice a month, but the urge to splurge is becoming much less as I feel the incredible rewards of my diet.

Other activities during my day include hiking with my two black labs, walking a lot, meditating (morning and evening), and giving thanks.

What I have described here is, of course, the Paleo Diet I've referred to throughout this book. If you look up the Paleo Diet, you'll find there are different ideas about it. Some say there is a lot of meat; raw, wild vegetables; and roots. However, cavemen did not have access to large supplies of meat, especially red meat. In fact, if you've ever been through survival training, you know how hard it is to come by meat in nature.

In the days of the caveman, there were sources of greens, herbs, roots, grains (not bread or cake), nuts, and berries. Storage was a problem, and much of the food was what we would call spoiled (nature's probiotics). Some of this natural spoilage became present-day foods like sauerkraut, pickles, wine, and beer.

It is the spirit of this diet that I want to propose. It is so logical. We are a product of millions of years of development into a being that is amazing. Along came extreme changes, just over the last few thousand years and especially over the last 100 years—and we expect to survive? Anyone giving any real thought to what has happened and why should be surprised not to see new epidemics of diseases popping up all around us.

As I mentioned earlier, I belong to an academy of physiology and benefit from exposure to the latest research on diet and health. There is now a worldwide pandemic of cirrhosis of the liver—due not to alcohol, but to the overconsumption of fructose sugar!

All these modern, convenient, delicious, "wholesome" treats modern science and industry are giving to us are killing us. Become informed!

What Can We Do to Overcome So Many Obstacles?

In my many years of counseling teenagers, I came up with a question that really got a strong reaction. I'd say, "Visualize that you're in a car heading through your life. Do you want to be in the backseat complaining about the driver going the wrong direction? Or are you willing to get into the driver's seat, take over the responsibilities, and drive your car of life where you want it to go?"

Most people spend more time planning this year's vacation than planning their life. Then they complain about the mess this neglect got them into or even blame it on others or on the government—then ask for help.

Let me suggest that we look at our lives as a beautiful painting, or as Dina Colman, author of Four Quadrant Living, puts it, the creation of our own masterpiece. Instead of letting everyday challenges own us and run our lives, let us take charge and direct that car of life to a beautiful place, creating a masterpiece to be proud of and being able to enjoy both looking back and looking forward.

To ensure the highest quality of life, one must be sure to plan in all four areas that influence that quality: your mental health and learning, your physical health, your social health, and your respect for all the many gifts you have been given on this earth.

To plan anything requires learning and understanding. Watching TV, playing video games, and reading meaningless literature may have some benefit, but they can also put you in that backseat of the car of life. Be sure to take time each day to learn a little about the four areas, even by walking and observing. You also have to plan your fun time.

Many of us made the decision to go into our career in our teens or twenties. If you don't like going to work today, it could be that the teenage you made a wrong decision. As Wayne Dyer said to a patient, you're fifty years old—would you go to an eighteen-year-old for advice on your future? If you're lucky and have the money, you might find it to be a beautiful, stress-relieving activity to begin to look at what you would really love doing and make plans to change.

In most cases, it is much too costly to change quickly. But just beginning to make plans to become what you most want to be can greatly change your stress level and increase your enjoyment of life. Many famous people did not start their successful career until their fifties— J.C. Penney, for one.

I am definitely not straying from the theme of this book. Never forget that your mental health can dominate your physical health and that it must be dealt with. Happiness is a fundamental part of healthiness. Perfect nutrition doesn't help if your stress hormones won't let you digest that food.

Now that we have a handle on our health and wellness, what are we to do about the greed and demagogy that have control of the health system? We must still turn to this system if bad luck strikes in the form of an injury, or if a friend or relative who doesn't have that handle on health needs medical care.

First, we must become informed on who and what to vote for and who and what to vote against. Demagogues will only listen if they are bribed, in one way or another, or if they fear losing their power. If those of us who want reform join large, well-funded groups, politicians will listen, as did Congress when Burzynski's patients demanded a hearing to stop the FDA and got it. This was a rather small but highly motivated group. Can you imagine what a well-organized group of millions of health-conscious voters could do?

Because I have had so many years of contact with people suffering needlessly, I tend to get overly emotional on the subject of health-care reform. It appears that since we can't beat them, we will have to join them. By this, I mean that all of us should join together to let those in power know just how powerful we are. A national, even worldwide, organization could be formed, wherein millions of small and large donations would make our leaders listen and clean up their act. If money and power are the only things that talk, this group could offer both.

We then would have the responsibility to keep politics and demagogy out of our organization. For some reason, which I touched on in the first chapter, whenever a number of people organize, someone wants to get political and take control. Proper organization and structure would be critical—and we must keep government out of it, just as I did when I started the Discovery Center. Because local people funded it and took part in the management of the center and the Discovery Thrift Shop, it is the only one of its kind, going stronger than ever after forty years.

It is my dream that such a nationwide organization might be created. We might call it the

People's Crusade for Health or United Health Advocates or any number of names. No matter what, something has to be done to stop the needless suffering. I invite everyone reading this book who's interested in working with me on this to contact me (see "About the Author" for contact information).

I wrote this book for the purpose of giving the average person a basic knowledge of what he or she needs in order to have more control over the quality of his or her health and health care. I tried very hard to emphasize the importance of becoming informed and knowledgeable.

I sincerely pray that I have accomplished these goals.

ABOUT THE AUTHOR

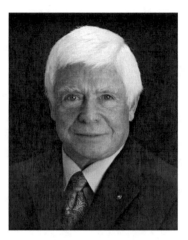

D
r. Robert J. Brown is director of the Advanced Oral Diagnostics and Treatment Center in Danville, California, where he specializes in temporomandibular joint dysfunction (TMJ), myofascial pain, and dental sleep medicine. He is passionate about teaching patients how to achieve optimal health, overcome and prevent disease, slow down the aging process, and understand the basis for true health.

Dr. Bob (as he's called by his patients) graduated from the University of California at Berkeley, where he majored in physiology and chemistry. He then attended the University of California Medical Center, graduating second in his class with a DDS specializing in orthodontics. His first orthodontics practice opened in 1964 in Walnut Creek, California.

Dr. Bob's interest in complementary and alternative medicine began in 1975, when he started studying homeopathy. Ten years later, he became a major consultant for Kaiser Hospitals in the fields of TMJ and myofacial pain syndrome. Memberships include the Foundation for Orthodontic Research, through which he promotes holistic health studies and introduced the concept of Zero Based Orthodontics, and the American Academy of Dental Sleep Medicine (AADSM). He is also on the board of directors of the School of Better Physiology, which teaches breathing to control blood oxygen and carbon dioxide, helping to regulate blood acidity and optimal oxygen levels.

Many civic organizations and services have benefited from Dr. Bob's leadership and guidance. He is the founding father of the Discovery Center, a successful center that provides services and support, including full-time psychologists, for places like foster homes for battered children and for people who are dealing with drug addiction—all at whatever price they can afford. He is founder of the San Ramon Valley youth council, which brings high school kids together to help build the community; president of the Danville Rotary Club; and founder of the first senior citizens' "Dial a Ride" program. In 1977 he was named Rotarian of the Year for Northern California.

Dr. Bob is an avid outdoorsman who enjoys hunting, fishing, fly fishing, boating, scuba diving, and gold prospecting.

For more information, please visit Dr. Bob's website at: www.DrBrownWhy.com

To contact Dr. Bob or request a media kit, please e-mail: Info@DrBrownWhy.com